Management of
Pituitary Tumours:
A Handbook

For Churchill Livingstone

Senior Medical Editor: Miranda Bromage
Project Editor: Mark Lane
Project Controller: Mark Sanderson
Design Direction: Sarah Cape
Copy Editor: Graham Wild
Indexer: Nina Boyd

Management of
Pituitary Tumours:
A Handbook

EDITED BY

Michael Powell MA MB BS FRCS
Consultant Neurosurgeon
The National Hospital For Neurology and Neurosurgery
Queen Square
London, UK

Stafford L. Lightman MA MB BChir PhD FRCP
Professor of Medicine
University of Bristol
Bristol Royal Infirmary
Bristol, UK

 CHURCHILL
LIVINGSTONE

NEW YORK
EDINBURGH
LONDON
MADRID
SAN
FRANCISCO
AND
TOKYO
1996

CHURCHILL LIVINGSTONE
Medical Division of Pearson Professional Limited

Distributed in the United States of America by Churchill
Livingstone Inc., 650 Avenue of the Americas, New York,
N.Y. 10011, and by associated companies, branches and
representatives throughout the world.

First published 1996

ISBN 0–443–05214–X

British Library Cataloguing in Publication Data
A catalogue record for this book is available from the British
Library.

Library of Congress Cataloging in Publication Data
A catalog record for this book is available from the Library
of Congress.

Produced by Longman Group FE Ltd
Printed in Singapore

The
publisher's
policy is to use
**paper manufactured
from sustainable forests**

Contents

Contributors

M. A. Hall-Craggs MB BS MD MRCP FRCR
Consultant Radiologist, Magnetic Resonance Unit, The Middlesex
Hospital UCLHT, London, UK

N. Hirsch MB BS FRCA
Consultant Anaesthetist, The National Hospital for Neurology and
Neurosurgery, Queen Square, London, UK

D. A. Jewkes MB BS FRCAnaes
Consultant Anaesthetist, National Hospital for Neurology and
Neurosurgery, Queen Square, London, UK

M. R. Johnson MB BS MRCP
Senior Lecturer and Honorary Consultant in Reproductive Medicine,
Academic Department of Obstetrics and Gynaecology, Chelsea and
Westminster Hospital, London, UK

B. Kendall FRCR FRCP FRCS FFRRCSI (Hon)
Consultant Neuroradiologist, Middlesex and Royal Free Hospitals,
London, UK

E. R. Laws (Jr) MD FACS
Professor of Neurosurgery, Professor of Medicine, University of
Virginia, Charlottesville, Virginia, USA

A. Levy, PhD MRCP
Consultant Senior Lecturer in Medicine, University of Bristol, Bristol
Royal Infirmary, Bristol, UK

D. J. O'Halloran BSc MD MRCP
Consultant Physician/Endocrinologist, Cork University Hospital, Cork, Ireland

S. L. Lightman MA MB BChir PhD FRCP
Professor of Medicine, University of Bristol, Bristol Royal Infirmary, Bristol and Honorary Consultant in Endocrinology, The National Hospital for Neurology and Neurosurgery, Queen Square, London, UK

W. I. McDonald BMED Sc MB ChB PhD FRACP FRCP FRCOphth
Professor of Clinical Neurology, Institute of Neurology, Queen Square, London, UK

M. Powell MA MB BS FRCS
Consultant Neurosurgeon, The National Hospital For Neurology and Neurosurgery, Queen Square, London, UK

S. M. Shalet MD FRCP
Professor of Endocrinology, Christie Hospital, Withington, Manchester, UK

W. K. 'Kling' Chong BMedSc MD MRCP FRCR
Consultant Neuroradiologist, Great Ormond St. Hospital for Children, London, UK

Acknowledgements

The authors are grateful for the editorial assistance provided by Dr Jennifer Shields and to Si Reichlin for his constructive criticism which was of great help to the editors in finalizing the shape of this book.

Introduction

Michael Powell, Stafford Lightman

We have written this handbook of the management of pituitary tumours primarily for the trainee in the specialties that treat these disorders. We have set out to make it 'user friendly' and not too complex. We would hope that the specialist already regularly treating pituitary disease will find the book helpful in keeping abreast of the advances in therapy in the allied fields. We give the view of the joint pituitary clinic at the National Hospital, Queen Square, where we have found that joint consultation between an endo-crinologist, a neurosurgeon, a neurologist and a radiotherapist gives an optimal, balanced approach to treatment plans. Every clinic is a discussion forum for each case, where all treatment modalities can be discussed, both between the doctors and the patient.

A pituitary clinic of this type centralizes the treatment of patients. This centralization of care is vital to improving quality of outcome. Not only does it ensure rapid clarification of diagnosis as in borderline Cushing's disease and acromegaly, but also assures the most appropriate treatment with mini-mum delay and morbidity. Pituitary surgery is a highly specialized art. It would be preferable if microsurgery for a microadenoma were only per-formed in centres that see in the region of 50 or more new cases per year. In skilled hands outcome is excellent. The disadvantage of pituitary surgery performed by surgeons with limited experience is increased morbidity and occasional mortality. The defence unions in the UK alone have at least one

1

case per year processing through the medicolegal system. Also associated with inexperience is a higher failure rate in terms of endocrine outcome together with an increased incidence of hypopituitarism and its attendant need for long-term hormone replacement.

Cost comparisons between specialist and general units should not be an issue for individual patients. By the end of treatment, specialist unit costs are probably less and definitely no greater than those of patients with poor outcomes requiring ongoing treatment because of unskilled management. In well-organized units, most endocrine investigations can be carried out on an outpatient or day case inpatient basis. Inpatient admission for surgery in a skilled centre is brief. In our unit this is usually less than seven days, with care streamlined to the needs of the pituitary patient. A prolactinoma or simple acromegalic microadenoma patient who has been appropriately investigated prior to admission is usually discharged within three or four days of surgery. This occurs in approximately three-quarters of all microadenoma patients.

Pituitary tumours make up 12.5% of intracranial tumours, but an average general practice will only expect to see one new case in every five to ten years and may have only two or three cases on their list in total. Recent epidemiological data suggest that there are approximately 1300 new cases of pituitary adenoma per year in the UK, not all of whom will need surgery. A single neurosurgeon in the UK would expect to see, on average, no more than two to four cases per year. We believe that the UK needs no more than six centres for pituitary microsurgery, each of which would see 100–150 cases per year. This would provide the necessary expertise for the optimal surgical treatment of all pituitary patients in the country.

Sadly, we have to accept that these idealized management arrangements are unlikely to be in place in the foreseeable future. Health care politics and local health trust economics are not favourable for the development of specialist centres, and small patient populations in some areas such as the Republic of Ireland simply could not justify them. Finally, the independant nature of the clinician and the 'interest' in unusual cases makes referral to another centre disappointingly unpopular. Hopefully this book will help clarify why these prejudices need to be reconsidered.

HISTORICAL PERSPECTIVES

The pituitary gland is an organ which has fascinated scientists and clinicians for centuries. The ancient Greeks believed that the pituitary removed waste products from the brain and secreted them as nasal mucus from the nose. There was remarkably little advance on this notion until the revolutionary discovery in the early 1930s of the neurosecretion of vasopressin and oxytocin from the posterior pituitary gland, and the demonstration of the prime importance of the anterior gland in the regulation of reproduction. It was a decade later that Geoffrey Harris and John Green suggested that nerve fibres in the hypothalamus secreted substances into the portal capillaries whence they were carried to the pituitary gland to excite or inhibit the activity of specialized secreting cells. After centuries of belief that it was a secretory organ, it had become the 'conductor of the endocrine orchestra' and subsequently, and more accurately, an amplifier for messages sent by the real conductor, the hypothalamus.

The first hypothalamic releasing factor, thyrotrophin releasing hormone, was finally characterized by Roger Guillemin and Andrew Schally in 1971, rapidly followed by other releasing factors. In 1977, the Nobel Prize for Medicine was awarded to them in recognition for this work. Since then, the identification of many other hypothalamic releasing and inhibitory factors has continued and to date almost 30 neuropeptides have been localized in the endocrine hypothalamus with neuroendocrine or neurotransmitter effects on hypothalamohypophyseal regulation. The CIBA Foundation has recently published an up-to-date review of this field, which we would recommend (*Functional Anatomy of the Neuroendocrine Hypothalamus*, CIBA Foundation Symposium 168, 1992, John Wiley).

Harvey Cushing stands as a giant in the history of pituitary disease. The founder of modern neurosurgery (in his surgical work, pioneering one of the transsphenoidal routes to the pituitary fossa) and a brilliant neurophysiologist, he made full and detailed descriptions of acromegaly and, of course, demonstrated the connection between the disease that bears his name and pituitary adenomas. Less well known, he also suggested that a patient with postpartum amenorrhoea and persistent lactation might be secreting a lactogenic hormone, which has now been identified as prolactin.

Since Cushing's day, pituitary management has benefited significantly from a number of technological advances in three main fields: firstly in endocrinology from radioimmunoassay, which has led to the the early diagnosis of disease caused by microadenomas and allowed us to assess the therapeutic value of the different treatments of the diseases; secondly, advances in computer imaging, initially with transmission computed tomography and now magnetic resonance imaging, have allowed anatomical diagnosis of microadenomas at a very early stage. Finally, the enormous improvements in surgical technique with the use of the operating microscope and microinstruments have allowed surgeons to make good use of both these techniques.

The history of the surgical management of pituitary disease starts, other than anecdotally, at the turn of the century. The first unsuccessful attempt to remove a pituitary tumour was made in 1889 by Sir Victor Horsley, who went on to perform a series of 10 such operations between 1904 and 1906. The first partial removal of pituitary tumour via the transsphenoidal approach was in 1907 by Schloffer. Surgeons such as Hirsch in Vienna, and Cushing in Boston, experimented with transsphenoidal surgery via the nasal and sublabial routes, although this was largely abandoned. We must admire their bravery in attempting their pioneering approaches with poor anaesthesia, lighting and lack of magnification, but not be surprised that for a long time radiotherapy held the centre ground in terms of useful treatment.

In the UK, the interest in transsphenoidal surgery was rekindled after the Second World War, when hypophysectomy was used as endocrine control of the spread of hormone-sensitive secondary cancers, such as breast and prostate. As neurosurgery was developing in other directions at that time, otolaryngologists such as Angel James in Bristol, Richards in Cardiff and Williams in London developed the transethmoidal technique, gaining enormous experience at a time when the endocrinologists were able to measure accurately and to a certain extent control pituitary diseases medically. It was only on the Continent and in Canada, through the legacy of Cushing's trainees (curiously from a Scot, Norman Dott who taught Guiott in Paris who taught Jules Hardy in Montreal), that transsphenoidal surgery remained in the neurosurgical domain.

The interest in radiation treatment to the pituitary gland began after Carl Beck (1905) described the positive treatment results with the use of Roentgen rays in 'Basedow's syndrome'. Two French physicians working separately, Gramegna and Beclere, extended this work to the management of acromegaly associated with the 'acidophil' pituitary tumour in 1909. Over the succeeding 20 years, several reports confirmed the value of radiotherapy in the management of pituitary tumours. With the major advances in megavoltage equipment and other developments in medical physics, the superiority of high-energy X-rays and particle irradiation compared with the lower-energy orthovoltage modalities, which were used in the early part of the century, have produced significant advantages in the field of radiotherapy to the pituitary gland.

Successful medical management of pituitary tumours is a much more recent therapeutic advance. The use of dopamine agonists in the 1970s and more recently the developement of somatostatin analogues have opened new non-invasive approaches to the treatment of pituitary tumours. This is clearly only the vanguard of new pharmacological approaches to pituitary disease.

The patho-physiology and pathogenesis of pituitary tumours

Andrew Levy, Stafford Lightman

Pituitary development
Theories of pathogenesis of pituitary adenomas
Cellular consequences of pituitary tumour formation
References

PITUITARY DEVELOPMENT

In early embryogenesis, cells destined to form the pituitary gland migrate medially from the ventral ridges of the primitive neural tube and are then pushed rostrally by the developing Rathke's pouch. After only 7 weeks of gestation the primitive pituitary cells are isolated from the stomadeum by the completion of the sella floor and from that time on, under the influence of the hypothalamus and a series of permissive and specific trans-acting proteins (only one of which, Pit 1, is currently well defined),[1,2] pituitary hormone genes are sequentially activated and their products translated and eventually secreted.[3,4] By the end of gestation the pituitary has developed into a complex and highly ordered structure which nevertheless retains considerable plasticity[5] and by the end of life, if histological examination of unselected autopsy material is to be believed, adenomas are present in as many as one in five.[6–8]

Cellular differentiation

Pituitary adenomas are for the most part benign epithelial tumours which develop from adenohypophyseal parenchymal cells, and as such their structure resembles normal pituitary histology to a greater or lesser extent. Fortunately, although tissue invasion at the microscopic level is thought to occur in over 40% of pituitary adenomas,[9] direct macroscopic invasion is rare.

Characterization of the normal cellular components of the pituitary and thus the identification of all potentially transformable pituitary target cells, which is clearly a prerequisite for the comprehensive analysis of tumours that arise from them, has not in practice proven easy to carry out. Close immunocytochemical scrutiny (not well supported at the level of gene expression) suggests that cells storing thyrotrophin and the gonadotrophins tend to lie medially with lactotrophs and somatotrophs more laterally, while adrenocorticotrophin-storing cells are distributed predominantly over the anterior and anterolateral surface of the gland. Clusters of folliculostellate cells form a network of interconnecting channels between the cords of secretory cells[10] and around them run the peptide-permeable capillaries that constitute the hypothalamohypophyseal portal system. In addition, a short portal system delivers venous blood to the anterior pituitary from the pars nervosa and in some individuals there may also be a small direct input from the systemic vasculature.[11]

Throughout this framework are scattered null cells—possibly pluripotent progenitor cells,[12,13] oncocytes,[14] stem cells,[15] cells derived from the remnants of Rathke's pouch,[16,17] a few immune cells, suggesting a low level of celllular immune response,[18] and cells secreting or co-secreting a number of peptides and hypothalamic hormones including vasoactive intestinal polypeptide (VIP),[19,20] growth hormone-releasing hormone (GRH) and somatostatin (SRIH),[21-25] corticotrophin-releasing hormone (CRH), galanin,[26-28] chorionic gonadotrophin,[29] substance P,[30] renin, pro-renin and cathepsin B,[31] transforming growth factor alpha (TGFα),[32] interleukin 6 (IL-6),[33] insulin-like growth factor 1 (IGF-1),[34] keratin, vimentin,[35] neuromedin B,[36,37] parathyroid hormone-related protein[38,39] and fibroblast growth factor (FGF).[40,41] The list of peptides known to be released by the pituitary[42,43] attests to the functional complexity of the structure.

Pituitary tumour classification

Although useful clinically, classifications of pituitary cells based on the immutable activation of one or two hormone genes are oversimplifications. Not only do adenomas arise from cells that were either never able to—or are no longer able to—secrete hormones, but multiple hormone gene and hormone receptor gene products are commonly identified in both native pituitary cells[44] and pituitary adenomas. This apparent lack of specificity of

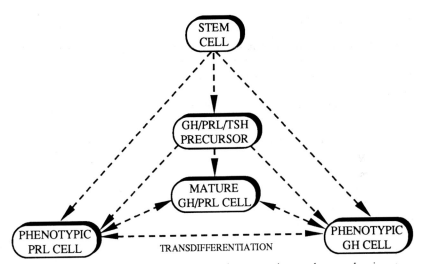

Fig. 1.1 Putative somatotroph and lactotroph maturation pathways showing transdifferentiation: the potential for direct change from one mature phenotype to another without dedifferentiation or stem cell proliferation.

gene expression as evinced, for example, by growth hormone (GH) gene expression in 50% of prolactinomas and 30% of corticotroph adenomas[45–47] is further complicated by the observation of rapid changes in the proportion of different cell types in the adult pituitary without a matching increase in mitotic figures. This strongly suggests that in the mature pituitary gland, transdifferentiation—a direct change from one fully differentiated phenotype to another—such as from lactotroph to somatotroph[48] or gonadotroph to lactotroph (during lactation for instance) can occur (Fig. 1.1). The production of bihormonal cells by syncytial fusion of different types has also been suggested[44] and compound tumours, such as those composed of adenohypophyseal and Rathke's pouch elements, have been described.[49] More confounding still is evidence that the phenotype of pituitary cells is determined at least in part by local environmental factors;[50] in other words, it may not be what a cell is that determines where it ends up in the pituitary gland, but where it is that determines what it becomes and how it is to behave.[51,52]

Attempts to classify pituitary parenchymal cells by analysing hypothalamic releasing hormone receptor activity, which might at first sight appear to be clinically highly relevant, have also foundered owing to the apparent promiscuity of receptor expression as shown by inositol phospholipid turnover and intracellular calcium ion fluctuations in response to hypothalamic hormones.[53–55] At the present time, therefore, the most clinically relevant classifications depend on tumour size and hormone secretion (even though many co-secretions and co-localizations have been recorded),[44,56–63] refined in many cases by analysis of the patterns of peptides hormone storage.

Further classifications based on cellular compositions, growth pattern and staining affinity, granularity, histological and electron microscopic appearances are also occasionally referred to.[64] As new hypothalamic hormone analogues become available, tumour classification may need further revision to encompass not only the features recognized for routine diagnosis, but also their complement of receptors and second messenger responses, so that specific chemotherapeutic targets can be identified and exploited.

THEORIES OF PATHOGENESIS OF PITUITARY ADENOMAS

Because the cells involved in adenoma formation may be derived from monoclonal or polyclonal expansions and may have phenotypes that are not only difficult to determine, but change during tumour development, it is not surprising that the pathogenesis of pituitary tumours remains for the most part a subject of speculation and debate. Broadly speaking, the potential mechanisms of oncogenesis can be grouped into: (1) abnormalities of genes regulating growth and development; (2) abnormalities of tumour suppressor genes which normally inhibit growth and proliferation; and (3) functional alterations in the genes controlling programmed cell death.

Excessive trophic hormone action

GRH[65-69] and CRH[70,71] have developmental and trophic as well as secretory effects, and GRH receptors and the response to GRH are not downregulated by continuous exposure to the peptide (Fig. 1.2 (1)). The evidence that thyrotrophin-releasing hormone (TRH) is trophic is considerably weaker, as (for example) true adenoma formation in hypothyroidism is very rare[72,73] and there is no evidence that under normal circumstances continual exposure to hypothalamic gonadotrophin-releasing hormone (GnRH) has any trophic action on gonadotrophs, although an indirect gonadotroph-dependent trophic effect on lactotrophs and corticotrophs has been suggested.[42,74] Paracrine and autocrine effects of hypothalamic releasing hormones—which may differ in local concentration and pattern of release—may not necessarily be the same, however, and the observation that a number of hypothalamic hormones (including VIP,[19] SRIH,[25] GRH[22] and TRH[75]) are made by the pituitary itself has fuelled speculation about their part in causation. Cell clusters containing high levels of CRH, oxytocin, GRH, TRH and/or SRIH transcripts are found in many pituitary adenomas, but for reasons that are so far obscure tend to predominate in somatotroph adenomas[25,76] (see Figs 1.3 and 1.4).

In favour of a primary hypothalamic aetiology for pituitary adenomas is the observation that paradoxical responses to exogenous glucose[77] and TRH[78] that are features of somatotroph adenomas also occur in vivo in cases caused by GRH-secreting adenomas, and that treatment of the latter abolishes the abnormal responses.[79] Also in favour of a primary hypo-

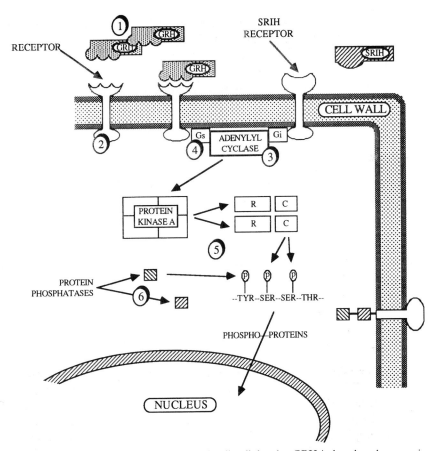

Fig. 1.2 Schematic diagram of a somatotroph cell wall showing GRH-induced nuclear protein phosphorylation. Interaction of ligand (1) with receptor (2) activates adenylyl cyclase (3) via the GTP binding protein Gs (4). Cyclic AMP cleaves protein kinase A into receptor and catalytic subunits (5), and the latter phosphorylates specific residues on proteins that, in addition to other actions, stimulate cell growth and division. If the phosphoproteins are not dephosphorylated by cytoplasmic and membrane-bound protein phosphatases (6), the proteins are free to be transported across the nuclear membrane where they directly influence DNA transcription.

thalamic pathology are the very rare cases of profound and prolonged hypo-thyroidism and hypogonadism in which true pituitary thyrotroph and gonadotroph adenomas arise.[80,81] Other extrinsic mechanisms, such as the development of a systemic blood supply depriving certain areas of the pituitary of dopamine-containing portal blood, predisposing to prolactinoma formation, have also been suggested.[11] Against a primary hypothalamic pathology in the majority of pituitary tumours is the low frequency of tumour recurrence post-operatively, the relatively low incidence of hyperplastic changes in 'target' cells adjacent to adenomas (21% of corticotroph and

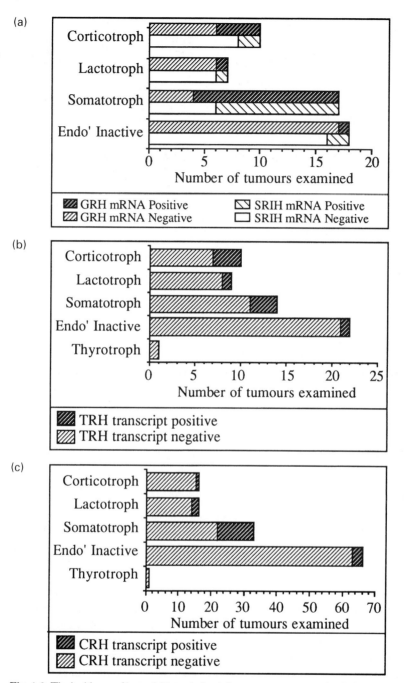

Fig. 1.3 The incidence of 'ectopic' hypothalamic hormone gene expression by human pituitary adenomas.

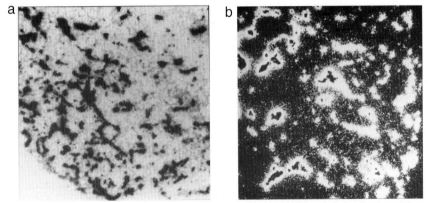

Fig. 1.4 Autoradiographs of adjacent sections of a somatotroph adenoma hybridized to probes complementary to CRH- (**a** bright field) and oxytocin- (**b** dark field) transcripts. In addition to GH transcripts (not shown), this tumour from an acromegalic patient can be seen to contain large amounts of (co-localized) CRH and oxytocin transcripts.

40% of somatotroph adenomas compared to 13% of normal pituitary glands)[82] and an increasing body of evidence to suggest that pituitary tumours are predominantly monoclonal in origin (see below).

Although a great deal of emphasis is currently being placed on the results of analysis of pituitary adenoma clonality, it should be noted that the strategy used[83] can only provide information in a small proportion of adenomas. These are derived from female patients who are heterozygotic for polymorphisms in specific X-linked genes, such as the hypoxanthine phosphoribosyl transferase (HPRT) gene and the phosphoglycerate kinase (PGK) gene. Even in these, the results may be frankly misleading if the HPRT and PGK sites are extensively methylated and, at its best, the method relies on the consistency of DNA recovery and probe hybridization to membrane-bound DNA that has previously been subjected to sequential restriction enzyme digestions. For technical reasons, experimental results are biased towards monoclonality, and as the development of a monoclonal pituitary adenoma does not exclude the participation of a number of early predisposing events, such as inappropriate hypothalamic hormone action or inappropriate receptor transcription culminating in monoclonal expansion, the classication of pituitary adenomas on this basis may not be as useful as would first appear. It is also possible that the final development of a monoclonal expansion of secreting cells might suppress surrounding hyperplasia present at an earlier stage of tumour induction.

The summated findings of studies from five different groups[84–88] show that all of the eight endocrinologically inactive adenomas, two gonadotroph adenomas, three somatotroph adenomas and a mammosomatotroph adenoma analysed were monoclonal. Two of the six lactotroph adenomas examined and the single plurihormonal adenoma were apparently polyclonal, but were thought to be contaminated with normal pituitary tissue, and of the 22 corticotrophs examined 17 were monoclonal, including, interestingly enough, five of the six tumours recovered from patients with Nelson's syndrome.

Receptor abnormalities

Paradoxical hormone responses, such as an increase in GH secretion or intracellular Ca^{2+} concentration in somatotroph adenomas in response to TRH,[89] VIP,[90,91] CRH,[92,93] GnRH and vasopressin,[53] are widely recognized, but the potential trophic implications of these observations are rarely addressed (Fig. 1.2 (2)). Widespread expression of multiple hypothalamic releasing hormone receptors in pituitary adenomas is complicated by the identification of quite different responses to ligands in what appear to be adenomas of similar origin. Some endocrinologically inactive adenomas, for example, have an inositol phospholipid turnover response to GnRH, but also increased inositol phospholipid turnover and intracellular Ca^{2+} levels in response to a pure GnRH antagonist.[55] Others respond to the agonist or antagonist alone.[55]

An abnormal complement of receptors caused by the failure to suppress apparently inappropriate hypothalamic hormone receptor gene expression in adenomatous pituitary cells might also be augmented by exogenous receptor-like molecules. It has been suggested, for instance, that part of the cytopathic effect of cytomegalovirus may be related to signalling system subversion, as the cytomegalovirus genome contains a number of sequences with considerable homology to those coding for G protein-coupled receptors.[94,95] If one or more of these became constitutively active during evolution, the trophic behaviour of an infected cell might be influenced.[94]

It is possible that growth factors such as the epidermal growth factor receptor may be involved in pituitary tumour formation.[96,97] This appears to be the case in astrocytomas, glioblastomas,[98,99] gliomas[100] and gastric cancer.[101] As distinct receptor functions such as the feedback inhibition and stimulation of mitogenesis can be selectively eliminated by single base changes,[102,103] a mutation leading to increased mitogenic stimulation is easy to envisage.

G protein malfunction

G proteins play a central role in signal transduction across the cell membrane. The α subunit, which dissociates from the β and γ subunits of heterotrimeric Gs when GTP displaces its bound GDP (Fig. 1.5), stimulates adenylyl cyclase to produce cyclic AMP from ATP. Cyclic AMP activates cyclic AMP-dependent protein kinases, increases intracellular Ca^{2+} and may also modify the activity of inositol phospholipid-dependent protein kinases and vice versa.[104] The weak intrinsic GTPase activity of $Gs\alpha$, potentiated

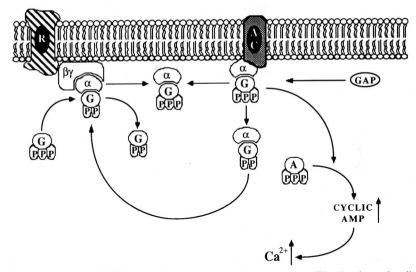

Fig. 1.5 Cartoon of GTPase activity. Activation of the receptor (R) stimulates the displacement of GDP by GTP on the α subunit of GTPase. The α subunit–GTP complex is cleaved from the βγ subunits of the heterotrimer and interacts with membrane-bound adenylyl cyclase (AC). Activated adenylyl cyclase stimulates cyclic AMP production from ATP and the increase in intracellular AMP produces a concomitant increase in intracellular Ca^{2+} levels, leading to hormone secretion and cell growth etc. The activity of the α subunit–GTP complex is turned off by its own intrinsic GTPase activity, by the GTPase activity of adenylyl cyclase and by GTPase activating protein (GAP). Liberated α subunit GDP reassociates with the βγ subunits and awaits the next activation cycle.

by the action of GAPs (GTPase-activating peptides, such as p120 GAP neurofibromin[105] and adenylyl cyclase itself[106,107]) dissociates GTP from Gsα and terminates the response. Guanine nucleotide-releasing or exchange molecules 'shuffle' the guanine nucleotides attached to G proteins with guanine nucleotides in intracellular stores, and as cellular GTP is generally at a higher molar concentration than GDP they tend to potentiate the action of Gs rather than terminate it.[108]

In addition, the presence of adenylyl cyclase isozymes[109,110] (Fig. 1.2 (3)) suggests that changes or mutations of adenylyl cyclase itself could alter the half-life of activated Gsα. As these signalling systems transduce messages that tell cells to grow and divide, changes in the intrinsic activity of any of their components[111] may predispose to adenoma formation. Specific examples of this in human pituitary adenomas are the two single point mutations in the Gsα subunit of GTPase, either of which results in constitutive activation of adenylyl cyclase (Figs 1.2 (4) and 1.5). These mutations are responsible for the formation of about 40% of somatotroph adenomas.[112–115] In tumours in which one of these mutations is present, sella morphology is more often normal than in somatroph adenomas arising from other causes, suggesting that Gs mutant-containing adenomas tend to be smaller.[115,116] There is as yet no general agreement about the relative secretory activity of these tumours. The *ras* protooncogenes (also involved in cell proliferation and differentiation)[117] are structurally related to the G protein family, and although the typical tumour-associated *ras* mutations have not been identified in pituitary adenomas, a change in the *H-ras* gene (Gly to Val) to codon 12 in a highly invasive prolactinoma has been described.[118]

Alterations in protein kinases

In addition to cyclic AMP-dependent and inositol phospholipid-dependent protein kinases, many receptors, such as the GH, IGF-1 and epidermal growth factor (EGF) receptors are either directly associated with or have intrinsic serine, threonine and/or tyrosine kinase activity (Fig. 1.2 (5)). Inappropriate activity of protein kinases or the phosphatases that terminate their effect (some of which are themselves receptor associated)[119] could disturb the duration of trophic signals and potentially lead to adenoma formation (Fig. 1.2 (6)).[120] As the cytopathogenic effect of a number of viruses may be related to their ability to introduce new or disturb the integrity of native protein kinases,[121,122] an association between pituitary adenoma formation and viral infection is possible, but is as yet unproven.

Local production of growth factors

In addition to fibroblast growth factor (FGF),[40,41] TGFα,[32] IGF-1[34] and hypothalamic releasing hormones, pooled serum-free conditioned medium from somatotroph and endocrinologically inactive adenoma cell cultures appears to contain a number of factors that stimulate [^{3}H]-thymidine uptake into cell lines.[41] Epidermal growth factor (EGF), TGF (which inhibits prolactin gene transcription in GH3 (rat mammosomatotroph adenoma-derived cells),[123] TGFε,[124] FGF and pituitary-derived mammary growth factor[125,126] have all been isolated from normal human pituitary. EGF has been shown to stimulate lactotroph proliferation and prolactin secretion from normal rat anterior pituitary cells, and in normoprolactinaemic women the TRH-induced increase in circulating prolactin is associated with suppression of serum EGF levels.[127] EGF receptors have not, however, been demonstrated in prolactinomas or in other pituitary adenomas.[96,97] Thus there is no evidence at present of a place for intrinsic growth factor expression in pituitary adenoma formation. Dramatic lactotroph hyperplasia in a strain of mice transgenic for an expression cassette in which nerve growth factor cDNA is driven by the prolactin promoter suggests, however, that it would be premature to discount such an association completely.

Anomalous vascular supply

There is speculation that the development of a systemic vascular supply could wash out hypothalamohypophyseal portal blood from areas of the anterior pituitary and so prevent dopamine and SRIH from reaching their target cells. It has been proposed that this mechanism may be responsible for the predisposition of Fischer 344 rats to lactotroph hyperplasia and prolactinoma formation in response to oestrogen treatment.[11] The same may also be true of releasing factors reaching the anterior pituitary from the neurohypophysis via the short portal system,[129,130] but as yet there is no direct evidence for this mechanism.

Tumour suppressor gene mutation

There is now good evidence that deletion or inactivation of tumour suppressor genes such as P53, Rb and DCC ('deleted in colonic carcinoma') predispose to human tumour formation.[131-136] Mutation of the p53 gene, for example, which codes for a protein that under normal circumstances prevents replication until the integrity of the genome has been assured,[137,138] is the most common genetic alteration found in human tumours. Under normal circumstances, if repair cannot be effected, sequestration of transcription factors by P53 protein is followed by activation of apoptosis.[139]

In addition to the allelic loss of chromosome 17p13 (the region coding for p53) in pituitary carcinomas, a series of other typical genomic changes have been found to cluster in central nervous system neoplasms, such as chromosome 10 monosomy in 28 of 29 glioblastomas, chromosome 17 losses in grade II astrocytomas[140] and amplification of normal or deletion mutations of the EGF receptor. Loss of heterozygosity of the MEN (multiple endocrine neoplasia) 1 tumour suppressor gene, which maps to chromosome 11q13, has been found in two of three prolactinomas examined.[141,142a] P53 mutation in the domain associated with 98% of P53-associated malignancies of the colon, lung, oesophagus, breast, liver, central nervous system and reticuloendothelial system (exons 4–8) were not, however, detected in DNA extracted from 29 randomly selected pituitary adenomas in our own studies (unpublished data).[142b]

Failure of programmed cell death

Until the importance of programmed cell death during development and as a regulator of turnover and remodelling of mature tissue was recognized, the possibility that tumour formation might result from 'the abnormal absence of cell death' was largely ignored. It is now known that inactivation of genes directly involved in the death pathway, such as P53,[139] can lead to tumour formation by failing to induce apoptosis if genomic integrity cannot be restored after induction of replication arrest. Overactivity of genes which act as 'antidotes to death', such as BCL-2, a mitochondrial and membrane protein, may have similar effects.

Conclusion

A number of the mechanisms described above probably need to act in concert to induce pituitary tumour formation. Inactivation of p53 or Rb by sequestration, or tyrosine kinase activation by the formation of complexes with viral antigens, intrinsic tyrosine/serine protein phosphatase activity or signalling system subjugation by other viruses, perhaps makes infection one of a number of possible predisposing events in the multistep progression towards pituitary adenoma formation. Changes in the level of trophic hormones, abnormal receptor expression and enhanced growth factor production further increase the responsiveness and instability of pituitary cells so that a single protooncogene hit, on, for example, one of the genes encoding proteins involved in the regulation of the cyclic AMP second messenger transduction pathway, will be sufficient to deregulate growth and result in monoclonal adenoma formation.

CELLULAR CONSEQUENCES OF PITUITARY TUMOUR FORMATION

Failure of appropriate hormone secretion from normal pituitary tissue adjacent to a developing pituitary tumour probably results from a number of mechanisms. These include disruption of normal cellular relationships and paracrine interactions, changes in systemic and hypothalamic–hypophyseal blood supplies, and conceivably 'transdifferentiation pressure' directly altering the identity of surrounding cells. Failure of the normal pituitary (or for that matter alteration in the contour of the sella) by 'direct compression' seems conceptually to be rather unlikely. The finding of inappropriately large circulating levels of one or sometimes two pituitary hormones is one of the most characteristic features of functioning pituitary adenomas, and gives rise to the classical symptoms and signs of hormone excess

Somatotroph adenomas

GH-secreting somatotroph adenomas are usually macroadenomas at diagnosis and frequently contain prolactin (PRL) (and sometimes thyrotrophin (TSH) transcripts and protein in addition to GH. Excessive secretion of hormones other than GH, which occurs in so-called monomorphous plurihormonal mammosomatotroph and bimorphous mixed somatotroph–lactotroph adenomas is, however, unusual.[143] Studies of intracellular calcium ion fluctuations and hormone secretion in response to various ligands show that somatotroph adenomas frequently have second messenger-coupled receptors for α and β adrenoceptors, activin A,[144] TRH,[145] vasopressin,

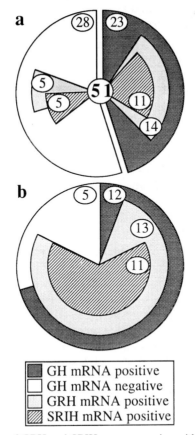

Fig. 1.6 The association of GRH and SRIH gene expression with GH gene expression in pituitary tumours (a) and with GH secretion and clinical acromegaly (b).

GnRH, insulin, SRIH,[146] arginine, dopamine,[146] oestradiol[97,147,148] and CRH. A familiar but nonetheless curious observation is that stimulation of these receptors with TRH,[78,149,150] GnRH or CRH[92,93] often induces paradoxical GH secretion, which like the typical GH secretory response to glucose has been exploited to form the basis of the diagnostic tests for somatotroph adenomas. Unexpectedly, the GH secretory response to GRH that is of course characteristic of normal somatotrophs is far from universal in somatotroph adenomas.[151] Whether this pattern of response is the result of 'inappropriate' trans-activating protein transcription, the loss of trans-acting proteins that normally suppress inappropriate transcription of receptors, or a combination of the two, is not yet known.

Many somatotroph adenomas have been found to express (or to contain subsets of cells that express) hypothalamic releasing hormone genes. Indeed expression of the GRH and SRIH genes appears to be associated with GH gene expression (Fig. 1.6a) and with clinical acromegaly (Fig. 1.6b).[25,76]

The possible aetiological significance of this finding is weakened, however, by the observation that CRH gene activity also seems to occur predominantly in somatotroph adenomas, with 33% of 33 somatotroph adenomas positive by in situ hybridization histochemistry, as opposed to only 13% of 16 prolactinomas, 6% of 16 corticotroph adenomas and 5% of 66 endocrinologically inactive adenomas.[152] TRH gene activity does not seem to have any greater specificity for somatotroph than for any other type of pituitary adenomas.

Corticotroph adenomas

The diagnostic tests used to distinguish the presence of secreting corticotroph adenomas from other causes of excessive hyperadrenocorticalism exploit the observation that unlike somatotroph adenomas, which are characterized by paradoxical responses, adenomatous corticotrophs retain many of the secretory responses of normal corticotrophs. Thus while the diurnal rhythm of adrenocorticotrophic hormone (ACTH) secretion and the rise in cortisol and GH in response to hypoglycaemia are diminished or lost, the feedback inhibitory effects of glucocorticoids are still present, although diminished, and the secretory response to an intravenous bolus of CRH is exaggerated.[153] A paradoxical ACTH secretory response to TRH[154] (blocked by the 5-hydroxytryptamine antagonist cyproheptadine)[155] occurs in about 30%, however, and a rise in prolactin in addition to ACTH and cortisol is often seen in response to CRH.[156] Many corticotroph adenomas also bear second messenger-coupled receptors for vasopressin and GnRH.[153]

Prolactinomas

The great majority of prolactinomas continue to express functional dopamine receptors which when stimulated result not only in an acute and persistent decrease in prolactin synthesis and secretion[157,158] but also in a reduction in lactotroph size and numbers.[159,160] The reason why some prolactinomas fail to respond to dopamine agonists is not understood, but is presumably related to a qualitative or quantitative change in dopamine receptors, or uncoupling of the receptors from second messenger pathways. Prolactinomas also express oestradiol receptors which when stimulated tend to stimulate prolactin transcription and secretion, and stimulate lactotroph proliferation.[97] Both basal and TRH-stimulated prolactin levels are abnormally high in prolactinomas (an effect that can sometimes be downregulated by prior treatment with thyroid hormones)[161] and although SRIH has no effect on prolactin levels in young females, the secretion of prolactin from mammosomatotroph adenomas is often reduced.[162] In addition to TRH, GnRH has also been found to increase inositol phospholipid turnover in the majority of prolactin transcript-containing adenomas in vitro,[53,163] and GnRH-associated peptide (a 56 amino acid peptide from the carboxyl terminal region (14–69) of the GnRH precursor)[164] has also been shown to release prolactin from pituitary adenomas.[165] Carcinomas of lactotrophs have been described but are very rare.[166–168]

Thyrotroph adenomas

Thyrotroph-secreting pituitary adenomas are relatively insensitive to the inhibitory effects of thyroid hormone feedback but are sensitive to the inhibitory effects of SRIH analogues which, at least in the short term, are used in their medical management.[81,169,170] As they progress, they become unresponsive to the stimulatory effects of TRH, and completely insensitive to the inhibitory effects of thyroid hormones and SRIH, both of which normally inhibit TSH secretion.[54,171] In many cases circulating TSH levels are within the normal range (i.e., not appropriately suppressed in response to the raised levels of circulating thyroid hormones), and in 80% intact TSH is accompanied by free α subunit secretion. Thyrotroph adenomas composed of two distinct cell types, one producing α subunit and another co-secreting α subunit and TSH, have been identified.[172] The co-secretion of GH and/or prolactin with TSH from thyrotroph adenomas has also been described[173] and is perhaps not surprising as the interaction of the pituitary-specific transactivator Pit 1 (which is present in thyrotrophs) with the GH and prolactin genes has to be specifically blocked to give the normal thyrotroph phenotype. Failure of this mechanism would facilitate inappropriate GH and prolactin transcription in thyrotrophs.

Gonadotroph and endocrinologically inactive adenomas

For reasons that are obscure, relatively few pituitary adenomas derived from the gonadotroph lineage secrete bioactive gonadotrophs. Radioimmunoassay and immunocytochemistry show that approximately 24% of macroadenomas in males produce and secrete dissociated α- or β-glycoprotein hormone subunits.[174,175] The majority of gonadotroph adenomas increase inositol phospholipid turnover and intracellular Ca^{2+} levels in vitro in response to TRH, GnRH[163] and GnRH analogues.[55] Administration of the same ligands as intravenous boluses in vivo results in secretion of glycoprotein hormone subunits in a significant proportion.[176] Gonadotroph adenomas have also been shown to variably express SRIH and dopamine receptors[177–179] although the application of long-acting SRIH analogues, dopamine agonists and GnRH analogues in clinical practice has not been particularly encouraging.[180,181] Gonadotrophin-secreting carcinomas of the pituitary have not been reported.

Endocrinologically inactive adenomas continue to present a clinical problem as their failure to secrete (by definition) makes their trophic responses to various ligands and the identify of the cells from which they originate difficult to determine in vivo. Many tumours originally described as non-functioning or endocrinologically inactive are now known to transcribe glycoprotein hormone subunits in variable amounts and have been discussed above. Others transcribe or transcribe and translate but do not secrete a variety of pituitary, placental and hypothalamic hormones,[20,76,182] and even these often contain proteins associated with secretory vesicles such as chromogranin and secretogranin[14,183,184] which are sometimes appropriately upregulated by GnRH.[185] Second to silent gonadotroph adenomas, silent corticotroph adenomas, transcribing proopiomelanocortin and often containing ACTH peptide, form the most well-defined group of apparently functionless adenomas.[186–189] Silent somatotroph adenomas almost certainly occur but are rare.[190]

In conclusion the unambiguous clinical classification of tumours based on the effects of excessive circulating hormones and immunocytochemical analysis of resected material is of limited value at the cellular and molecular level. Functional GRH receptors, for example, which one would expect to find on somatotroph adenoma cell membranes, are present in only a minority of cases. TRH, GnRH and vasopressin receptors, which might be expected to be limited to specific adenoma subtypes, are widely expressed by somatotroph, corticotroph and lactotroph adenomas as well as by many 'endocrinologically inactive' pituitary tumours. Similarly, studies of hormone gene expression show that many tumours transcribe (but do not necessarily translate) hormone genes apparently equally indiscriminately. Thus, however appealing it is to classify tumours morphologically, such categorization may obscure the presence of targets against which new clinical interventions could be directed. It is salutary to remember that as exciting as the discovery of the gsp oncogene was in contributing to the explanation of the pathogenesis of pituitary adenomas (and more recently the McCune–Albright syndrome),[191] it only accounts for the formation of a minority of cases of one subtype of secreting adenoma. This remains a very challenging area for the cell biologist and endocrinologist which will undoubtably result in the generation of much exciting new data over the next decade.

REFERENCES

1. Ingraham HA, Chen R, Mangalam HJ et al. A tissue-specific transcription factor containing a homeodomain specifies a pituitary phenotype. Cell 1988; 55: 519–529.
2. Mangalam HJ, Albert VR, Ingraham HA et al. A pituitary POU domain protein, Pit-1, activates both growth hormone and prolactin promoters transcriptionally. Genes Dev 1989; 3: 946–948.
3. Baker BL, Jaffe RB. The genesis of cell types in the adenohypophysis of the human fetus as observed with immunocytochemistry. Am J Anat 1975; 143: 137–162.
4. Aubert ML, Grumbach MM, Kaplan SL. The ontogenesis of human fetal hormones. III. Prolactin. J Clin Invest 1975; 56: 155–164.
5. Krishnan KRR, Doraiswamy PM, Lurie SN et al. Pituitary size in depression. J Clin Endocrinol Metab 1991; 72: 256–259.
6. Costello RT. Subclinical adenoma of the pituitary gland. Am J Pathol 1936; 12: 205–216.

7. Molitch ME, Russell EJ. The pituitary 'incidentaloma'. Ann Intern Med 1990; 112: 925–931.
8. Kontogeorgos G, Kovacs K, Horvath E, Scheithauer BW. Multiple adenomas of the human pituitary: a retrospective autopsy study with clinical implications. J Neurosurg 1991; 74: 243–247.
9. Sautner D, Saeger W. Invasiveness of pituitary adenomas. Pathol Res Pract 1991; 187: 632–636.
10. Baes M, Allaerts W, Denef C. Evidence for functional communication between folliculo-stellate cells and hormone-secreting cells in perifused anterior pituitary cell aggregates. Endocrinology 1987; 120: 685–691.
11. Elias KA, Weiner RI. Direct arterial vascularization of estrogen-induced prolactin-secreting anterior pituitary tumors. Proc Natl Acad Sci USA 1984; 81: 4549–4553.
12. Kovacs K, Horvth E, Ryan N, Ezrin C. Null cell adenoma of the human pituitary. Virchows Arch 1980; 387: 165–174.
13. Kontogeorgos G, Horvath E, Kovacs K, Killinger DW, Smyth HS. Null cell adenoma of the pituitary with features of plurihormonality and plurimorphous differentiation. Arch Pathol Lab Med 1991; 115: 61–64.
14. Lloyd RV, Jin L, Fields K et al. Analysis of pituitary hormones and chromogranin A mRNAs in null cell adenomas, oncocytomas, and gonadotroph adenomas by in situ hybridization. Am J Pathol 1991; 139: 553–564.
15. Shiino M, Ishikawa H, Rennels EG. Specific subclones derived from a multipotential clone of rat anterior pituitary cells. Am J Anat 1978; 153: 81–95.
16. Ishikawa H, Shiino M, Arimura A, Rennels EG. Functional clones of pituitary cells derived from Rathke's pouch epithelium of fetal rats. Endocrinology 1977; 100: 1227–1230.
17. Nakasu S, Nakasu Y, Kyoshima K, Watanabe K, Handa J, Okabe H. Pituitary adenoma with multiple ciliated cysts: transitional cell tumor? Surg Neurol 1989; 31: 41–48.
18. Rossi ML, Jones NR, Esiri MM, Havas L, al-Izzi M, Coakham HB. Mononuclear cell infiltrate and HLA-Dr expression in 28 pituitary adenomas. Tumori 1991; 76: 543–547.
19. Nagy G, Mulchahey JJ, Neill JD. Autocrine control of prolactin secretion by vasoactive intestinal peptide. Endocrinology 1988; 122: 364–366.
20. Hsu DW, Riskind PN, Hedley-Whyte ET. Vasoactive intestinal peptide in the human pituitary gland and adenomas: an immunocytochemical study. Am J Pathol 1989; 135: 329–338.
21. Pagesy P, Li JY, Rentier-Deirue Y, LeBouc Y, Martial JA, Peillon F. Evidence of pre-prosomatostatin mRNA in human normal and tumoral anterior pituitary gland. Mol Endocrinol 1989; 3: 1289–1294.
22. Peillon F, Le-Dafniet M, Garnier P et al. Neurohormones coming from the normal and tumoral human anterior pituitary: secretion and regulation in vitro. Pathol Biol (Paris) 1989; 37: 840–845.
23. Joubert DB, Benlot C, Lagoguey A et al. Normal and growth hormone (GH)-secreting adenomatous human pituitaries release somatostatin and GH-releasing hormone. J Clin Endocrinol Metab 1989; 68: 572–577.
24. Wakabayashi I, Inokuchi K, Hasegawa O, Sugihara H, Minami S. Expression of growth hormone (GH)-releasing factor gene in GH-producing pituitary adenoma. J Clin Endocrinol Metab 1992; 74: 357–361.
25. Levy A, Lightman SL. Relationship between somatostatin and growth hormone messenger ribonucleic acid in human pituitary adenomas: an in situ hybridization histochemistry study. Clin Endocrinol 1989; 32: 661–668.
26. Vrontakis ME, Sano T, Kovacs K, Friesen HG. Presence of galanin-like immunoreactivity in nontumorous corticotrophs and corticotroph adenomas of the human pituitary. J Clin Endocrinol Metab 1990; 70: 747–751.
27. Hsu DW, Hooi SC, Hedley-Whyte ET, Strauss RM, Kaplan LM. Coexpression of galanin and adrenocorticotropic hormone in human pituitary and pituitary adenomas. Am J Pathol 1991; 138: 897–909.
28. Sano T, Vrontakis ME, Kovacs K, Asa SL, Friesen HG. Galanin immunoreactivity in neuroendocrine tumors. Arch Pathol Lab Med 1991; 115: 926–929.
29. Hammond E, Griffin J, Odell WD. A chorionic gonadotropin-secreting human pituitary cell. J Clin Endocrinol Metab 1991; 72: 747–754.

30. Roth KA, Krause JE. Substance-P is present in a subset of thyrotrophs in the human pituitary. J Clin Endocrinol Metab 1990; 71: 1089–1095.
31. Saint-Andre JP, Rohmer V, Pinet F, Rousselet MC, Bigorgne JC, Corvol P. Renin and cathepsin B in human pituitary lactotroph cells: an ultrastructural study. Histochemistry 1989; 91: 291–297.
32. Kudlow JE, Bjorge JD. TGF alpha in normal physiology. Semin Cancer Biol 1990; 1: 293–302.
33. Jones TH, Justice S, Price A, Chapman K. Interleukin-6 secreting human pituitary adenomas in vitro. J Clin Endocrinol Metal 1991; 73: 207–209.
34. Alberti VN, Takita LC, de-Mesquita MI, Percario S, Maciel RM. Immunohistochemical demonstration of insulin-like growth factor I (IGF-1) in normal and pathological human pituitary glands. Pathol Res Pract 1991; 187: 541–542.
35. Ogawa A, Sugihara S, Hasegawa M et al. Intermediate filament expression in pituitary adenomas. Virchows Arch B 1990; 58: 341–349.
36. Jones MP, Withers DJ, Ghatei MA, Bloom SR. Evidence for neuromedin-B synthesis in the rat anterior pituitary gland. Endocrinology 1992; 130: 1829–1836.
37. Minamino N, Kangawa K, Matsuo H. Neuromedin B is a major bombesin-like peptide in rat brain: regional distribution of neuromedin B and neuromedin C in rat brain, pituitary and spinal cord. Biochem Biophys Res Commun 1984; 124: 925–932.
38. Kitazawa S, Fukase M, Kitazawa R et al. Immunohistological evaluation of parathyroid hormone-related protein in human lung cancer and normal tissue with newly developed monclonal antibody. Cancer 1991; 67: 984–989.
39. Davidson LA, McNicol AM. Localization of parathyroid hormone related protein immunoreactivity in the human pituitary gland and in pituitary adenomas. J Endocrinol Invest 1991; 14 suppl 4–6: 205.
40. Silverlight JJ, Prysor-Jones RA, Jenkins JS. Basic fibroblast growth factor in human pituitary tumours. Clin Endocrinol (Oxf) 1990; 32: 669–676.
41. Webster J, ten Horn CD, Bevan JS, Ham J, Scanlon MF. Preliminary characterisation of growth factors secreted by human pituitary tumours. J Endocrinol Invest 1991; 14 suppl 4–6: 207.
42. Denef C, Tilemans D, Andries M. Paracrine control of cell mitosis of lactotrophs, somatotrophs and corticotrophs by growth factors secreted by gonadotrophs in the immature rat adenohypophysis. J Endocrinol Invest 1991; 14 suppl 4–6: 19.
43. Paulssen RH, Paulssen EJ, Alestrom P, Gordeladze JO, Gautvik KM. Specific antisense RNA inhibition of growth hormone production in differentiated rat pituitary tumour cells. Biochem Biophys Res Commun 1990; 171: 293–300.
44. Newman GR, Jasani B, Williams ED. Multiple hormone storage by cells of the human pituitary. J Histochem Cytochem 1989; 37: 1183–1192.
45. Levy A, Lightman SL. Quantitative in-situ hybridization histochemistry of anterior pituitary hormone mRNA species in human pituitary adenomas. Acta Endocrinol (Copenh) 1988; 119: 397–404.
46. Saeger W, Uhlig H, Baz E, Fehr S, Ludecke DK. In situ hybridization for different mRNA in GH-secreting and in inactive pituitary adenomas. Pathol Res Pract 1991; 187: 559–563.
47. Kameya T, Furuhata S. Plurihormonal adenomas: analysis of 62 cases. Pathol Res Pract 1991; 187: 574–576.
48. Kineman RD, Faught WJ, Frawley LS. Steroids can modulate transdifferentiation of prolactin and growth hormone cells in bovine pituitary cultures. Endocrinology 1992; 130: 3289–3294.
49. Nishio S, Mizuno J, Barrow DL, Takei Y, Tindall GT. Pituitary tumors composed of adenohypophysial adenoma and Rathke's cleft cyst elements: a clinicopathological study. Neurosurgery 1987; 21: 371–377.
50. Alvarez-Vega P, Gil-Loyzaga P, Vaticon D, Esquifino Y, Tresguerres JAF. Parotid gland transplanted to the sella turcica after hypophysectomy is able to partially substitute pituitary function. J Endocrinol Invest 1991; 14 suppl 4–6: 82.
51. Snyder EY, Deitcher DL, Walsh C, Arnold-Aldea S, Hartwieg EA, Cepko CL. Multipotent neural cell lines can engraft and participate in development of mouse cerebellum. Cell 1992; 68: 33–51.
52. Renfranz PJ, Cunningham MG, McKay RDG. Region-specific differentiation of the

hippocampal stem cell line HiB5 upon implantation into the developing mammalian brain. Cell 1991; 66: 713–729.

53. Levy A, Lightman SL, Hoyland J, Mason WT. Inositol phospholipid turnover and intracellular Ca^{2+} responses to thyrotrophin-releasing hormone, gonadotrophin-releasing hormone and arginine vasopressin in pituitary corticotroph and somatotroph adenomas. Clin Endocrinol 1989; 33: 73–79.

54. Levy A, Eckland DJA, Gurnery AM, Reubi J-C, Doshi R, Lightman SL. Somatostatin and thyrotrophin-releasing hormone response and receptor status of a thyrotropin secreting pituitary adenoma. J Neuroendocrinol 1989; 1: 321–326.

55. Levy A, Lightman SL, Hoyland J, Rawlings S, Mason WT. A gonadotrophin-releasing hormone (GnRH) antagonist distinguishes three populations of GnRH analogue-responsive cells in human and rat pituitary in vitro and produces an acute increase in intracellular Ca^{2+} concentration without inducing gonadotropin secretion. Mol Endocrinol 1990; 4: 678–684.

56. Kovacs K, Horvath E, Asa SL, Stefaneanu L, Sano T. Pituitary cells producing more than one hormone: human pituitary adenomas. Trends Endocrinol Metab 1989; 1: 104–107.

57. Malarkey WB, Kovacs K, O'Dorisio TM. Response of a GH- and TSH-secreting pituitary adenoma to a somatostatin analogue (SMS 201-995): evidence that GH and TSH coexist in the same cell and secretory granule. Neuroendocrinology 1989; 49: 267–274.

58. Ambrosi B, Bassetti M, Ferrario R, Medri G, Giannattasio G, Faglia G. Precocious puberty in a boy with a PRL-, LH- and FSH-secreting pituitary tumour: hormonal and immunocytochemical studies. Acta Endocrinol (Copenh) 1990; 122: 569–576.

59. Hirasawa R, Hashimoto K, Makino S et al. Effect of a long-acting somatostatin analogue (SMS 201-995) on a growth hormone and thyroid stimulating hormone-producing pituitary tumor. Acta Med Okayama 1991; 45(2): 107–115.

60. Berg KK, Scheithauer BW, Felix I et al. Pituitary adenomas that produce adrenocorticotropic hormone and alpha-subunit: clinicopathological, immunohistochemical, ultrastructural, and immunoelectron microscopic studies in nine cases. Neurosurgery 1990; 26: 397–403.

61. Kamijo K, Sato M, Saito T et al. An ACTH and FSH producing invasive pituitary adenoma with Crooke's hyalinization. Pathol Res Pract 1991; 187: 637–641.

62. Mahler C, Verhelst J, Klaes R, Trouillas J. Cushing's disease and hyperprolactinemia due to a mixed ACTH- and prolactin-secreting pituitary macroadenoma. Pathol Res Pract 1991; 187: 598–602.

63. Bermingham J, Haenel LC. Hyperthyroidism with an FSH- and TSH-secreting pituitary adenoma. J Am Osteopath Assoc 1989; 89: 1560–1566.

64. Kovacs K, Horvath E. Pathology of pituitary tumours. In: Molitch ME (eds) Pituitary tumours: diagnosis and management. Philadelphia: Saunders 1987; pp 529–551.

65. Cella SG, Locatelli V, Mennini T et al. Deprivation of growth hormone-releasing hormone early in the rat's neonatal life permanently affects somatotropic function. Endocrinology 1990; 127: 1625–1634.

66. Wehrenberg WB, Bloch B, Phillips BJ. Antibodies to growth hormone-releasing factor inhibit somatic growth. Endocrinology 1984; 115: 1218–1220.

67. Asa SL, Scheithauer BW, Bilbao JM et al. A case for hypothalamic acromegaly: a clinicopathological study of six patients with hypothalamic gangliocytomas producing growth hormone-releasing hormone. J Clin Endocrinol Metab 1984; 58: 796–803.

68. Burton FH, Hasel KW, Bloom FE, Sutcliffe JG. Pituitary hyperplasia and gigantism in mice caused by a cholera toxin transgene. Nature 1991; 350: 74–77.

69. Struthers RS, Vale WW, Arias C, Sawchenko PE, Montminy MR. Somatotroph hypoplasia and dwarfism in transgenic mice expressing a non-phosphorylatable CREB mutant. Nature 1991; 350: 622–624.

70. Gertz BJ, Contreras LN, McComb DJ, Kovacs K, Tyrrell JB, Dallman MF. Chronic administration of corticotropin-releasing factor increases pituitary corticotroph number. Endocrinology 1987; 120: 381–388.

71. Stenzel-Poore MP, Cameron VA, Vaughan J, Sawchenko PE, Vale W. Development of Cushing's syndrome in corticotropin-releasing factor transgenic mice. Endocrinology 1992; 130: 3378–3386.

72. Katz MS, Gregerman RI, Horvath E, Kovacs K, Ezrin C. Thyrotroph cell adenoma of

the human pituitary gland associated with primary hypothyroidism: clinical and morphological features. Acta Endocrinol (Copenh) 1980; 95: 41–48.

73. Wajchenberg BL, Tsanaclis AM, Marino J. TSH-containing pituitary adenoma associated with primary hypothyroidism manifested by amenorrhoea and galactorrhoea. Acta Endocrinol (Copenh) 1984; 106: 61–66.

74. Tilemans D, Andries M, Denef C. Luteinizing hormone-releasing hormone and neuropeptide Y influence deoxyribonucleic acid replication in three anterior pituitary cell types: evidence for mediation by growth factors released from gonadotrophs. Endocrinology 1992; 130: 882–894.

75. Pagesy P, Croissandeau G, Le Dafniet M, Peillon F, Li JY. Detection of thyrotropin-releasing hormone (TRH) mRNA by the reverse transcription-polymerase chain reaction in the human normal and tumoral anterior pituitary. Biochem Biophys Res Commun 1992; 182: 182–187.

76. Levy A, Lightman SL. Growth hormone-releasing hormone transcripts in human pituitary adenomas. J Clin Endocrinol Metab 1992; 74: 1474–1476.

77. Caplan RH, Koob L, Abellera RM, Pagliara SA, Kovacs K, Randall RV. Cure of acromegaly by operative removal of an islet cell tumor of the pancreas. Am J Med 1978; 64: 874–882.

78. Irie MT, Sushima T. Increase in serum growth hormone concentration following thyrotropin-releasing hormone injection in patients with acromegaly or gigantism. J Clin Endocrinol Metab 1972; 35: 97–100.

79. Sassolas G, Chayvialle JA, Partensky C et al. Acromégalie, expression clinique de la production de facteurs de libération de l'hormone de croissance (G.R.F.) par une tumeur pancréatique. Ann Endocrinol (Paris) 1983; 44: 347–354.

80. Gesundheit N, Petrick PA, Nissim M et al. Thyrotropin-secreting pituitary adenomas: clinical and biochemical heterogeneity. Ann Intern Med 1989; 111: 827–835.

81. Smallridge RC. Thyrotrophin-secreting pituitary tumors. In: Molich ME (eds) Endocrinology and metabolism clinics of North America. Philadelphia: Saunders 1987; pp 765–792.

82. Saeger W, Lüdecke DK. Pituitary hyperplasia: definition, light and electron microscopical structures and significance in surgical specimens. Virchows Arch A 1983; 399: 277–287.

83. Vogelstein B, Fearon ER, Hamilton SR, Preisinger AC, Willard HF, Michelson AM, Riggs AD, Orkin SH. Clonal analysis using recombinant DNA probes from the X-chromosome. Cancer Res 1987; 47: 4806–4813.

84. Alexander JM, Biller BMK, Bikkai H, Zervas NT, Arnold A, Klibanski A. Clinically nonfunctioning pituitary tumors are monoclonal in origin. J Clin Invest 1990; 86: 336–340.

85. Herman V, Fagin J, Gonsky E, Ezrin C, Kovacs K. Clonal origins of pituitary adenomas. J Clin Endocrinol Metab 1990; 71: 1427–1433.

86. Jacoby LB, Hedley-Whyte ET, Pulaski K, Seizinger BR, Martuza RL. Clonal origin of pituitary adenomas. J Neurosurg 1990; 73: 731–735.

87. Schulte HM, Oldfield EH, Allolio B, Katz DA, Berkman RA, Ali IU. Clonal composition of pituitary adenomas in patients with Cushing's disease: determination by X-chromosome inactivation analysis. J Clin Endocrinol Metab 1991; 73: 1302–1308.

88. Gicquel C, LeBouc Y, Craig I, Luton JP, Girard F, Bertagna X. Pituitary corticotroph adenomas are monoclonal. Atlanta, Georgia: 1991; 439.

89. Molitch ME. Acromegaly. In: Collu R, Brown GM, Van Loon GR (eds) Clinical neuroendocrinology. Boston: Blackwell, 1988; 189–227.

90. Matsushita N, Kato Y, Katakami H, Shimatsu A, Yanaihara N, Imura H. Stimulation of growth hormone release by vasoactive intestinal polypeptide from human pituitary adenomas in vitro. J Clin Endocrinol Metab 1981; 53: 1297–1300.

91. Kato Y, Shimatsu A, Matsushita N, Ohta H, Imura H. Role of vasoactive intestinal polypeptide (VIP) in regulating the pituitary function in man. Peptides 1984; 5: 389–394.

92. Pieters GFFM, Hermus ARMM, Smals AGH, Kloppenborg PWC. Paradoxical responsiveness of growth hormone to corticotropin-releasing factor in acromegaly. J Clin Endocrinol Metab 1984; 58: 560–562.

93. Ishibashi M, Hara T, Tagusagawa Y et al. Effects of ovine corticotropin-releasing factor and hydrocortisone on growth hormone secretion by pituitary adenoma cells of acromegaly in culture. Acta Endocrinol (Copenh) 1984; 106: 443–447.

94. Ross EM. Viral hijack of receptors. Nature 1990; 344: 707–708.
95. Chee MS, Satchwell SC, Preddie E, Weston KM, Barrell BG. Human cytomegalovirus encodes three G protein-coupled receptor homologues. Nature 1990; 344: 774–777.
96. Birman P, Michard M, Li JY, Peillon F, Bression D. Epidermal growth factor-binding sites, present in normal human and rat pituitaries, are absent in human pituitary adenomas. J Clin Endocrinol Metab 1987; 65: 275–281.
97. Peillon F, Le-Dafniet M, Garnier P, Brandi AM, Moyse E, Birman P, Blumberg-Tick J, Grouselle D, Joubert-Bression D. Receptors and neurohormones in human pituitary adenomas. Horm Res 1989; 31(1–2): 13–18.
98. Burgart LJ, Robinson RA, Haddad SF, Moore SA. Oncogene abnormalities in astrocytomas: EGF-R gene alone appears to be more frequently amplified and rearranged compared with other protooncogenes. Mod Pathol 1991; 4: 183–186.
99. Reifenberger G, Prior R, Deckert M, Wechsler W. Epidermal growth factor receptor expression and growth fraction in human tumours of the nervous system. Virchows Arch A Pathol Anat 1989; 414: 147–155.
100. Humphrey PA, Gangarosa LM, Wong AJ, Archer GE, Lund-Johansen M, Bjerkvig R, Laerum OD, Friedman HS, Bigner DD. Deletion-mutant epidermal growth factor receptor in human gliomas: effects of type II mutation on receptor function. Biochem Biophys Res Commun 1991; 178: 1413–1420.
101. Lemoine NR, Jain S, Silvestre F et al. Amplification an overexpression of the EGF receptor and c-erbB-2 proto-oncogenes in human stomach cancer. Br J Cancer 1991; 64: 79–83.
102. Mohammadi M, Dionne CA, Li W et al. Point mutation in FGF receptor eliminates phophatidylinositol hydrolysis without affecting mitogenesis. Nature 1992; 358: 681–684.
103. Peters KG, Marie J, Wilson E et al. Point mutation of an FGF receptor abolishes phophatidylinositol turnover and Ca^{2+} flux but not mitogenesis. Nature 1992; 358: 678–681.
104. Gusovsky F, Gutkind JS. Selective effects of activation of protein kinase C isozymes on cyclic AMP accumulation. Mol Pharmacol 1991; 39: 124–129.
105. Li Y, Bollag G, Clark R et al. Somatic mutations in the neurofibromatosis 1 gene in human tumors. Cell 1992; 69: 275–281.
106. Arshavsky VY, Bownds MD. Regulation of deactivation of photoreceptor G protein by its target enzyme and cGMP. Nature 1992; 357: 416–417.
107. Bourne HR, Stryer L. The target sets the tempo. Nature 1992; 358: 541–543.
108. Shou C, Farnsworth CL, Neel BG, Feig LA. Molecular cloning of cDNAs encoding a guanine-nucleotide-releasing factor for Ras p21. Nature 1992; 358: 351–354.
109. Gao B, Gilman AG. Cloning and expression of a widely distributed (type IV) adenylyl cyclase. Proc Natl Acad Sci USA 1991; 88: 10178–10182.
110. Feinstein PG, Schrader KA, Bakalyar HA et al. Molecular cloning and characterization of a Ca^{2+}/calmodulin-insensitive adenylyl cyclase from rat brain. Proc Natl Acad Sci USA 1991; 88(22): 10173–10177.
111. Corven EJv, Groenink A, Jalink K, Eichholtz T, Moolenaar WH. Lysophosphatidate-induced cell proliferation: identification and dissection of signaling pathways mediated by G proetins. Cell 1989; 59: 45–54.
112. Vallar L, Spada A, Giannattasio G. Altered Gs and adenylate cyclase activity in human growth hormone-secreting pituitary adenomas. Nature 1987; 330: 566–568.
113. Landis CA, Masters SB, Spada A, Pace AM, Bourne HR, Vallar L. GTPase inhibiting mutations activate the α chain of Gs and stimulate adenylyl cyclase in human pituitary tumours. Nature 1989; 340: 692–696.
114. Lyons J, Landis CA, Harsh G et al. Two G protein oncogenes in human endocrine tumors. Science 1990; 249: 655–659.
115. Spada A, Arosio M, Bochicchio D et al. Clinical, biochemical, and morphological correlates in patients bearing growth hormone-secreting pituitary tumors with or without constitutively active adenylyl cyclase. J Clin Endocrinol Metab 1990; 71: 1421–1426.
116. Landis CA, Harsh G, Lyons J, Davis R L, McCormick F, Bourne HR. Clinical characteristics of acromegalic patients whose pituitary tumors contain mutant Gs protein. J Clin Endocrinol Metab 1990; 71: 1089–1095.
117. Barbacid M. Ras genes. Annu Rev Biochem 1987; 56: 779–827.

118. Karga HJ, Alexander JM, Hedley-Whyte ET, Klibanski A, Jameson JL. Ras mutations in human pituitary tumors. J Clin Endocrinol Metab 1992; 74: 914–919.
119. Streuli M, Krueger NX, Tsai AYM, Saito H. A family of receptor-linked protein tyrosine phosphatases in humans and *Drosophila*. Proc Natl Acad Sci USA 1989; 86: 8698–8702.
120. Banks P. Tyrosine phosphatases: cellular superstars in the offing. J NIH Res 1990; 2: 62–66.
121. Bautch VL, Toda S, Hassell JA, Hanahan D. Tissue specificity of oncogene action: endothelial cell tumours in polyoma middle T transgenic mice. IARC Sci Publ 1989; 96: 255–266.
122. Guan K, Broyles SS, Dixon JE. A Tyr/Ser protein phosphatase encoded by vaccinia virus. Nature 1991; 350: 359–362.
123. Delidow BC, Billis WM, Agarwal P, White BA. Inhibition of prolactin gene transcription by transforming growth factor-beta in GH3 cells. Mol Endocrinol 1991; 5: 1716–1722.
124. Halper J, Parnell PG, Carter BJ, Ren P, Scheithauer BW. Presence of growth factors in human pituitary. Lab Invest 1992; 66: 639–645.
125. Fernig DG, Smith JA, Rudland PS. Relationship of growth factors and differentiation in normal and neoplastic development of the mammary gland. Cancer Treat Res 1991; 53: 47–78.
126. Chomczynski P, Kuryl T, Brar A. Mitogenic effect of a factor from rat somatomammotrophs on mammary epithelial cells. Endocrinology 1992; 131: 228–234.
127. Chen CF, Kurachi H, Miyake A, Aono T, Tanizawa O. Suppression of serum immunoreactive human epidermal growth factor by acute increase in prolactin in women. Endocrinol Jpn 1989; 36: 203–209.
128. Borrelli E, Sawchenko PE, Evans RM. Pituitary hyperplasia induced by ectopic expression of nerve growth factor. Proc Natl Acad Sci USA 1992; 89: 2764–2768.
129. Hyde JF, Murai I, Ben-Jonathan N. The rat posterior pituitary contains a potent prolactin-releasing factor: studies with perifused anterior pituitary cells. Endocrinology 1987; 121: 1531–1539.
130. Hyde JF, Ben-Jonathan N. Characterization of prolactin-releasing factor in the rat posterior pituitary. Endocrinology 1988; 122: 2533–2539.
131. Wu SQ, Storer BE, Bookland EA et al. Nonrandom chromosome losses in stepwise neoplastic transformation in vitro of human uroepithelial cells. Cancer Res 1991; 51: 3323–3326.
132. Tanaka K, Oshimura M, Kikuchi R, Seki M, Hayashi T, Miyaki M. Suppression of tumorigenicity in human colon carcinoma cells by introduction of normal chromosome 5 or 18. Nature 1991; 349: 340–342.
133. Hollstein M, Sidransky D, Vogelstein B, Harris CC. p53 mutations in human cancers. Science 1991; 253: 49–53.
134. Malkin D, Li FP, Strong LC et al. Germ line p53 mutations in a fmailial syndrome of breast cancer, sarcomas, and other neoplasms. Science 1990; 250: 1223–1238.
135. Oliner JD, Kinzler KW, Meltzer PS, George DL, Vogelstein B. Amplification of a gene encoding a p53-associated protein in human sarcomas. Nature 1992; 358: 80–83.
136. Michalovitz D, Halevy O, Oren M. p53 mutations: gains or losses? J Cell Biochem 1991; 45: 22–29.
137. Farmer G, Bargonetti J, Zhu H, Friedman P, Prywes R, Prives C. Wild-type p53 activates transcription in vitro. Nature 1992; 358: 83–86.
138. Lane DP. p53, guardian of the genome. Nature 1992; 358: 15–16.
139. Yonish RE, Resnitzky D, Lotem J, Sachs L, Kimchi A, Oren M. Wild-type p53 induces apoptosis of myeloid leukaemic cells that is inhibited by interleukin-6. Nature 1991; 353: 345–347.
140. James CD, Carlbom E, Dumanski JP et al. Clonal genomic alterations in glioma malignancy stages. Cancer Res 1988; 48: 5546–5551.
141. Bystrom C, Larsson C, Blomberg C et al. Localization of the MEN 1 gene to a small region within chromosome 11q13 by deletion mapping in tumors. Proc Natl Acad Sci USA 1990; 87: 1968–1972.
142a. Bale AE, Norton JA, Wong EL et al. Allelic loss on chromosome 11 in hereditary and sporadic tumors related to familial multiple endocrine neoplasia Type 1. Cancer Res 1991; 51: 1154–1157.
142b. Levy A, Hall L, Kendall WA, Lightman SL. P53 Gene mutations in Pituitary Adenomas: Rare Events Clin Endocrinol 1994; 41: 809–14.

143. Asa SL, Kovacs K, Horvath E, Singer W, Smyth HS. Hormone secretion in vitro by plurihormonal pituitary adenomas of the acidophil cell line. J Clin Endocrinol Metab 1992; 75: 68–75.
144. Kitaoka M, Takano K, Tanaka Y, Kojima I, Teramoto A, Ogata E. Inhibition of growth hormone secretion by activin A in human growth hormone-secreting tumour cells. Acta Endocrinol Copenh 1991; 124: 666–671.
145. Garcia-Garcia J, Jimenez-Reina L, Barcia-Luna PP, Leal-Cerro A. In vitro short-term effects of SMS 201–995, bromocriptine and TRH on growth hormone cell morphology from human pituitary adenomas. Histol Histopathol 1989; 4: 223–233.
146. Sadoul JL, Thyss A, Freychet P. Invasive mixed growth hormone/prolatin secreting pituitary tumour: complete shrinking by octreotide and bromocriptine, and lack of tumour growth relapse 20 months after octreotide withdrawal. Acta Endocrinol Copenh 1992; 126: 179–183.
147. Ishibashi M, Yamaji T. Effects of hypophysiotropic factors on growth hormone and prolactin secretion from somatotroph adenomas in culture. J Clin Endocrinol Metab 1985; 60: 985–988.
148. Chiodini PG, Liuzzi A, Dallabonzana D, Oppizzi G, Verde G. Changes in growth hormone (GH) secretion induced by human pancreatic GHRH releasing hormone-44 in acromegaly: a comparison with thyrotropin-releasing hormone and bromocriptine. J Clin Endocrinol Metab 1985; 60: 48–52.
149. Faglia G, Beck-Peccoz P, Ferrari C, Travaglini P, Ambrosi B, Spada A. Plasma growth hormone response to thyrotropin-releasing hormone in patients with active acromegaly. J Clin Endocrinol Metab 1973; 36: 1259–1262.
150. Lamberts SWJ, Klijn JGM, van Vroonhoven CCG, Stefanko SZ. Different responses of growth hormone secretion to guanfacine, bromocriptine, and thyrotropin-releasing hormone in acromegalic patients with the pure growth hormone (GH) containing and mixed GH/prolactin containing pituitary adenomas. J Clin Endocrinol Metab 1985; 60: 1148–1153.
151. Dufy-Barbe L, Bresson L, Sartor P, Odessa M-F, Dufy B. Calcium homeostasis in growth hormone (GH)-secreting adenoma cells: effect of GH-releasing factor. Endocrinology 1992; 131: 1436–1444.
152. Levy A, Lightman SL. Corticotrophin-releasing hormone gene expression in human pituitary adenomas. Clin Endocrinol 1992; submitted for publication.
153. Findling JW, Kehoe ME, Shaker JL, Raff H. Routine inferior petrosal sinus sampling in the differential diagnosis of adrenocorticotropin (ACTH)-dependent Cushing's syndrome: early recognition of the occult ectopic ACTH syndrome. J Clin Endocrinol Metab 1991; 73: 408–413.
154. Krieger DT, Luria M. Plasma ACTH and cortisol responses to TRF, vasopressin or hypoglycaemia in Cushing's disease and Nelson's syndrome. J Clin Endocrinol Metab 1977; 44: 361–368.
155. Krieger DT, Condon EM. Cyproheptadine treatment of Nelson's syndrome: restoration of plasma ACTH circadian periodicity and reversal of response to TRF. J Clin Endocrinol Metab 1978; 46: 349–352.
156. Schulte HM, Allolio B, Günther RW et al. Selective bilateral and simultaneous catheterization of the inferior petrosal sinus: CRF stimulates prolactin secretion from ACTH-producing microadenomas in Cushing's disease. Clin Endocrinol 1988; 28: 285–295.
157. Hancock KW, Scott JS, Lamb JT, Gibson RM, Chapman C. Long term suppression of prolactin concentrations after bromocriptine induced regression of pituitary prolactinomas. Br Med J 1985; 290: 117–118.
158. Johnston DG, Prescott RWG, Kendall-Taylor P et al. Hyperprolactinemia: long-term effects of bromocriptine. Am J Med 1983; 75: 868–874.
159. McGregor AM, Scanlon MF, Hall K, Cook DB, Hall R. Reduction in size of a pituitary tumor by bromocriptine therapy. N Engl J Med 1979; 300: 291–293.
160. Landolt AM, Minder H, Osterwalder V, Landolt TA. Bromocriptine reduces the size of cells in prolactin-secreting pituitary adenomas. Experientia 1982; 39: 625–626.
161. DeLean AL, Ferland L, Drouin J, Kelly PA, Labrie F. Modulation of the pituitary thyrotropin releasing hormone receptor levels by estrogens and thyroid hormones. Endocrinology 1977; 100: 1496–1504.
162. Lamberts SWJ. The role of somatostatin in the regulation of anterior pituitary hormone

secretion and the use of its analogs in the treatment of human pituitary tumors. Endocr Rev 1986; 9: 417–436.

163. Levy A, Lightman SL. Effects of thyrotropin-releasing hormone and gonadotropin releasing hormone on inositol phospholipid turnover in endocrinologically inactive pituitary adenomas and prolactinomas. J Clin Endocrinol Metab 1989; 69: 122–126.

164. Nikolics K, Mason AJ, Szonyi E, Ramachandran J, Seeburg PH. A prolactin-inhibiting factor within the precursor for human gonadotropin-releasing hormone. Nature 1985; 316: 511–517.

165. Forget H, Lafond J, Collu R. Inhibition of prolactin release by gonadotropin-releasing hormone-associated peptide in benign, dopamine-sensitive and in malignant, dopamine-resistant pituitary tumours. J Neuroendocrinol 1992; 4: 59–62.

166. Scheithauer BW, Randall RV, Kramer S. Prolactin cell carcinoma of the pituitary: clinicopathologic, immunohistochemical and ultrastructural study of a case with cranial and extracranial metastases. Cancer 1985; 55: 598–604.

167. Martin NA, Hales M, Wilson CB. Cerebellar metastasis from a prolactinoma during treatment with bromocriptine. J Neurosurg 1981; 55: 615–519.

168. UHS, Johnson C. Metastatic prolactin-secreting pituitary adenoma. Hum Pathol 1984; 15: 94–96.

169. Warnet A, Lajeunie E, Gelbert F et al. Shrinkage of a primary thyrotropin-secreting pituitary adenoma treated with the long-acting somatostatin analogue octreotide (SMS 201–995). Acta Endocrinol (Copenh) 1991; 124: 487–491.

170. Chayen SD, Gross D, Makhoul O, Glaser B. TSH producing pituitary tumor: biochemical diagnosis and long-term medical management with octreotide. Horm Metab Res 1992; 24: 34–38.

171. Guillausseau PJ, Chanson PH, Timsit J et al. Visual improvement with SMS 201–995 in a patient with a thyrotropin-secreting pituitary adenoma. N Engl J Med 1987; 317: 53–54.

172. Terzolo M, Orlandi F, Bassetti M et al. Hyperthyroidism due to a pituitary adenoma composed of two different cell types, one secreting alpha-subunit alone and another cosecreting alpha-subunit and thyrotropin. J Clin Endocrinol Metab 1991; 72: 415–421.

173. Scheithauer BW, Horvath E, Kovacs K et al. Plurihormonal pituitary adenomas. Semin Diagn Pathol 1986; 3: 69–82.

174. Snyder PJ. Gonadotroph cell adenomas of the pituitary. Endocr Rev 1985; 6: 552–563.

175. Katznelson L, Alexander HM, Bikkal HA, Jameson JL, Hsu DW, Klibanski A. Imbalanced follicle-stimulating hormone β-subunit hormone biosynthesis in human pituitary adenomas. J Clin Endocrinol Metab 1992; 74: 1343–1351.

176. Snyder PJ, Sterling FH. Hypersecretion of LH and FSH by a pituitary adenoma. J Clin Endocrinol Metab 1976; 42: 544–550.

177. Vance ML, Ridgway EC, Thorner MO. Follicle-stimulating hormone- and alpha-subunit-secreting pituitary tumor treated with bromocriptine. J Clin Endocrinol Metab 1985; 61: 580–584.

178. Oppenheim DS, Klibanski A. Medical therapy of glycoprotein hormone-secreting pituitary tumors. Endocrinol Metab Clin North Am 1989; 18: 339–358.

179. Kwekkeboom DJ, Lamberts SWJ. Long-term treatment with the dopamine agonist CV205–502 of patients with a clinically non-functioning, gonadotroph, or α-subunit secreting pituitary adenoma. Clin Endocrinol 1992; 36: 171–176.

180. Roman SH, Goldstein M, Kourides IA, Comite F, Bardin CW, Krieger DT. The luteinizing hormone-releasing hormone (LHRH) agonist [D-Trp⁶-Pro⁹-NEt]LHRH increased rather than lowered LH and α-subunit levels in a patient with an LH-secreting pituitary tumor. J Clin Endocrinol Metab 1984; 58: 313–319.

181. Sassolas G, Lejeune H, Trouillas J et al. Gonadotropin-releasing hormone agonists are unsuccessful in reducing tumoral gonadotropin secretion in two patients with gonadotropin-secreting pituitary adenomas. J Clin Endocrinol Metab 1988; 67: 180–185.

182. Levy A, Lightman SL. Local production of hypothalamic trophic peptides in human pituitary tumours. Clin Chem Enzyme Commun 1992; in press.

183. Schmid KW, Kroll M, Hittmair A et al. Chromogranin A and B in adenomas of the pituitary: an immunocytochemical study of 42 cases. Am J Surg Pathol 1991; 15: 1072–1077.

184. Lloyd RV, Jin L, Song J. Ultrastructural localization of prolactin and chromogranin B

messenger ribonucleic acids with biotinylated oligonucleotide probes in cultured pituitary cells. Lab Invest 1990; 63: 413–419.

185. Song JY, Jin L, Chandler WF et al. Gonadotropin-releasing hormone regulates gonadotropin beta-subunit and chromogranin-B messenger ribonucleic acids in cultured chromogranin-A-positive pituitary adenomas. J Clin Endocrinol Metab 1990; 71: 622–630.

186. Horvath E, Kovacs K, Killinger DW, Smyth HS, Platts ME, Singer W. Silent corticotroph adenomas of the human pituitary gland; a histologic, immunocytologic and ultrastructural study. Am J Pathol 1980; 98: 617–638.

187. Horvath E, Kovacs K, Smyth HS et al. A novel type of pituitary adenoma: morphological features and clinical correlations. J Clin Endocrinol Metab 1988; 66: 1111–1118.

188. Kovaks K, Horvath E, Bayley TA, Hassaram ST, Ezrin C. Silent corticotroph cell adenoma with lysosomal accumulation and crinophagy: a distinct clinicopathological entity. Am J Med 1978; 64: 492–499.

189. Nagaya T, Seo H, Kuwayama A et al. Pro-opiomelanocortin gene expression in silent corticotroph-cell adenoma and Cushing's disease. J Neurosurg 1990; 72: 262–267.

190. Kineman RD, Faught WJ, Frawley LS. Bovine pituitary cells exhibit a unique form of somatotrope secreting heterogeneity. Endocrinology 1990; 127: 2229–2235.

191. Weinstein LS, Shenker A, Gejman PV, Merino MJ, Friedman E, Speigel A M. Activation mutations of the stimulatory G protein in the McCune–Albright syndrome. N Engl J Med 1991; 325: 1688–1695.

CHAPTER 2

The approach to the 'pituitary' patient: an overview

Stafford Lightman, Michael Powell

All patients
Microprolactinomas
Macroprolactinomas
Acromegaly
Cushing's adenomas
Non-secreting macroadenomas
Craniopharyngiomas
References

In the subsequent chapters, the many varied ways in which pituitary tumours can present will be described. These fall into three main categories:

1. Primary hormonal hypersecretion syndromes such as hyperprolactinaemia, acromegaly and Cushing's disease
2. Visual presentation; field and acuity defects and ophthalmoplegias
3. Non-specific presentations including infertility, headache, pituitary hypofunction, epilepsy and others.

Each patient requires an individual approach to investigation and management, although there are common themes to them all. We strongly suggest that it is appropriate to refer the patient to a specialist centre for definitive diagnosis and treatment at the earliest opportunity. It is important to realize that not all patients need full endocrinological, radiological and ophthalmological assessment. This would not only be an unnecessary waste of resources, but also some investigations such as the insulin stress test can be unpleasant and even dangerous in inexperienced centres.

ALL PATIENTS

Every patient will need a minimum of two hormone investigations—basal prolactin levels and thyroid function tests—and also good-quality magnetic resonance scanning (MRI). If unavailable, this could be investigated at a unit with a fourth-generation CT scanner where dynamic contrast fine-cut imaging can be carried out.

Thyroid function is of fundamental importance to the well-being of the patient. Although thyroid hypofunction is not particularly common in patients with pituitary adenomas, it is one of the most important to diagnose. Primary hypothyroidism can cause pituitary enlargement and hyperprolactinaemia. Whether primary or secondary, hypothyroidism will make surgical intervention dangerous until treated.

Prolactin levels are of crucial importance in all patients. Raised prolactin levels in the absence of treatment with dopamine antagonists, hypothyroidism or other factors which cause secondary hyperprolactinaemeia (see Ch. 3) should always indicate the need for pituitary imaging. Even relatively small increases in prolactin levels can indicate the presence of a non-functioning macroadenoma or other parasellar lesions which compress the pituitary stalk, reducing hypothalamic inhibitory control of prolactin release.

Imaging of pituitary lesions has been a contentious issue. There are those who would argue that not all patients require imaging, particularly for the patient with hyperprolactinaemia. However, not all of these have a prolactinoma, as non-functioning adenomas and other non-adenomatous sellar lesions can all present with raised levels. (Laws recently reports non-adenomatous parasellar lesions with prolactin levels in excess of 10,000 mg/ml.) These patients are not likely to do well on dopamine agonists, although the clinician may be misled by the return of normal endocrine function, such as with restoration of the menstrual cycle. If the clinician does not know what is being treated, the management is neither logical nor optimal.

There is no doubt that modern MRI is the radiological investigation of choice. It has the resolution to display the smallest of microadenomas, although not all. It will rule out the giant aneurysm, the worst fear of the transsphenoidal surgeon, as well as showing the details of the skull base which the surgeon will need to navigate to the fossa, whether via the sphenoid or the cranial approach. Sadly, the older machines do not have the resolution to show microadenomas and the skull base details will be insufficient for safe surgery. It is true that most, but crucially not all, of these features can be shown by a highly dedicated good-quality CT unit. However, these are costly in scanner time and require considerable skill. Vascular details are far less satisfactory, there is a small but appreciable dose of irradiation and not all patients can tolerate and hold the extended neck position required.

In the remainder of the chapter we will set out outlines for the minimum investigation for each common pituitary condition, although details will be given in greater depth in subsequent chapters.

MICROPROLACTINOMAS

Investigations

Thyroid function, prolactin and MRI are the only investigations needed. We believe that first-line treatment is medical.

Treatment

Dopamine agonist dosage is started at low levels and titrated against subsequent serum prolactin levels.

MACROPROLACTINOMAS

Investigations

Prolactin level, thyroid function and MRI are required as above. It is very unusual to need cortisol replacement in these patients, but if their symptoms are suggestive of hypopituitarism, such as weight loss and exhaustion, morning cortisol should be measured. If borderline, a synacthen test should be performed. Vital pre-treatment investigation will include ophthalmological review with visual field and acuity measurement.

Treatment

In our practice, the primary treatment of macroprolactinomas is with a dopamine agonist, as is the treatment of microadenomas. Although surgeons debate the relative merits of dopamine agonists, even the most aggressive surgeon would have to agree that surgery on a giant prolactinoma seldom normalizes the prolactin level and bromocriptine will almost inevitably be required long term. We would answer the debate by a typical example:

A 28-year-old woman presented with rapidly failing vision over a period of weeks. She had a four-year history of amenorrhoea and when admitted to hospital could barely navigate around the room. Vision was reduced to finger counting in a nasal hemifield in her best eye and only light appreciation

(a)   (b)

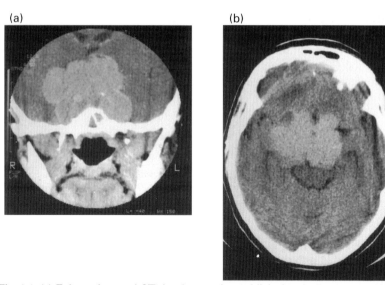

Fig. 2.1 **(a)** Enhanced coronal CT showing massive multilobed prolactinoma, engulfing carotids and extending to the third ventricle. **(b)** Axial enhanced CT above the level of the clinoids showing extent of the same tumour.

in the other. Figure 2.1 shows the CT scan from the referring hospital. This huge multilobular lesion is a formidable challenge to any surgeon, and if the prolactin level had not been in excess of 150,000 mg/ml the woman would have been submitted to difficult surgery, probably as a two-stage procedure, followed by radiotherapy, with little hope for significant improvement in her vision. As it was, on a small dose of bromocriptine her vision was virtually normal in both eyes within 48 h.

If a 'horrible' surgical case such as this does so well on bromocriptine, there is little justification for a surgical approach to the smaller and 'easier' macroprolactinomas without a dopemine agonist trial.

The patient *must* be reviewed at the end of one week of dopamine agonist therapy to ensure that the visual fields have not deteriorated. If within one month the visual fields have failed to improve and the prolactin levels not fallen by at least 50%, surgery is indicated. As noted above, surgery is seldom totally curative, although it should adequately decompress the chiasm.

ACROMEGALY

Diagnosis is the key. Many patients are discovered incidentally and often late.

Investigations

Growth hormone series and IGF1 levels with prolactin and thyroid function are required. Good MRI is essential.

Treatment

The primary treatment is surgical. It would be very unusual for a patient to be too unwell to undergo surgery with adequate preparation. Secondary treatment for failed surgery is with radiotherapy. Somatostatin therapy may be indicated whilst the hormone-reducing effects of radiotherapy are awaited, which may take several years. Dopamine agonist therapy may be helpful in mixed prolactin and GH-secreting tumours.

We see no place for the primary treatment of these tumours with somatostatin or its analogues. There is little evidence that these tumours usefully regress on this treatment, and the results and minor risks of surgery far outweigh any advantage of medical treatment, even in acromegalic macroadenomas.

CUSHING'S ADENOMAS

The key to the Cushing's patient is diagnosis, which is often very complex. It is vital to establish the primary cause of the disorder and it important to be aware that ectopic ACTH sources may cause considerable diagnostic problems. We would stress that all these patients should be referred to a specialist centre.

Investigation

Urinary free cortisol, the loss of diurnal cortisol rhythm and the lack of response to overnight dexamethasone suppression are the primary screening procedures. Fuller details are provided in detail in Chapter 3.

Treatment

The primary treatment is transsphenoidal surgery. Secondary treatment for failed pituitary surgery is adrenalectomy and pituitary irradiation.

NON-SECRETING MACROADENOMAS

These tumours usually present with visual disturbance but may on occasions present with headache or pituitary hypofunction. Although they usually require surgery, there are grounds for observing their progress with time.

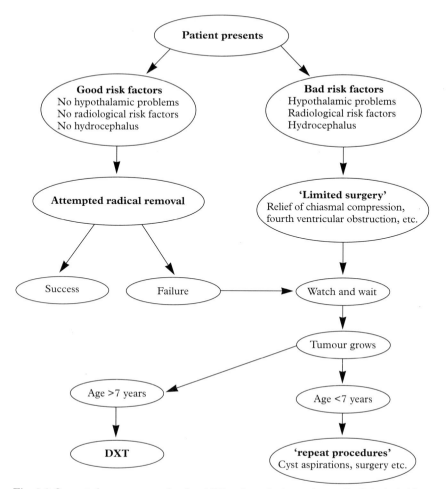

Fig. 2.2 Suggested management plan for childhood craniopharyngiomas. Radiological risk factors include involvement of structures above the chiasm, such as the hypothalamus as well as extensive lateral spread, particularly through the cavernous sinus and surrounding the carotid arteries. (After R. D. Hayward, personal communication.)

Investigation

Thyroid function, prolactin and MRI remain the essential prerequisites. Cortisol status should be assessed if there are signs of hypopituiarism or if surgery is to be delayed or not performed. All tumours that extend into the suprasellar recess require ophthalmological assessment.

Treatment

Surgery is usually needed. The place of radiotherapy is increasingly debated. We recommend it to prevent recurrence if there is residual tissue, although not always in the elderly nor in the younger patient if the post-operative scan is clear.

CRANIOPHARYNGIOMAS

These tumours are probably the most difficult of all parasellar tumours to manage, and how it is done remains controversial. The issues are discussed in some detail in the chapter 11. Centralizing the management of this problematic lesion is essential, particularly in the paediatric group. Adult tumours are often much more indolent than in children and may not require intervention. A flow chart of investigation and management is given in Figure 2.2.[1]

REFERENCES

1. Powell MP, Thompson D. The neurosurgical approach to hypothalamo-hypophyseal tumours. In: Brook CB, ed. Clinical paediatric endocrinology. Oxford: Blackwells, 1995: pp 346–357.

The medical management of pituitary tumours

Mark Johnson
Stafford L. Lightman

The majority of pituitary tumours are asymptomatic as shown by the discrepancy between the reported prevalance of 200 per million population[1] and the post-mortem findings of pituitary tumours in 10–27% of the population.[2,3] Those that present do so either because of local pressure effects, or as a result of the effects of hormone hypersecretion or hyposecretion. A combination of greater awareness of pituitary diseases coupled with the recent advances in imaging of the pituitary fossa has resulted in the relatively early diagnosis of pituitary tumours in most cases. Improvements in our diagnostic skills, however, have not been matched by advances in therapy, the foundations of which still rest on surgery and radiotherapy in all but the cases of prolactinoma and, arguably, acromegaly. In this chapter, we will consider the different modes of presentation, investigation and treatment of pituitary tumours.

PRESENTATION

Pituitary tumours may be classified as either functioning or endo crinologically inactive. Functioning tumours secrete exessive amounts of active hormones, while the endocrinologically inactive tumours either secrete no hormones at all or only secrete inactive hormones or hormone fragments. Pituitary tumours are also classified by virtue of their size into the arbitrary division of those less than 1 cm in diameter (microadenomas) and those greater than 1 cm (macroadenomas). These divisions together define the usual manner of tumour presentation. Microadenomas present with hormone hypersecretion, while macroadenomas more frequently compress and invade local structures with or without hormone hypersecretion. Thus, pituitary tumours may present with any combination of hormone deficiency, hormone excess or local invasion. The effects of tissue compression and/or invasion will be considered first, followed by the presentation of patients with hormone hypersecretion states.

Compression and invasion

Local structures may be invaded and destroyed by a pituitary tumour. An understanding of the anatomy of the pituitary gland is essential to appreciate the effect of an enlarging tumour and is described in detail in Chapter 6. In summary, the gland lies in the pituitary fossa of the sphenoid bone, covered by the diaphragma sellae and just below the optic chiasm. It is bordered on each side by the cavernous sinuses. It follows, therefore, that spread anteriorly and inferiorly invades the sphenoid sinus; lateral spread can result in invasion of the cavernous sinus with potential cranial nerve palsy and even temporal lobe epilepsy; and finally, and most commonly, spread superiorly results in stretching of the diaphragma which may cause frontal, temporal or retro-orbital headaches (most common in acromegaly), but, more seriously, the optic chiasm is compressed resulting in acuity and visual field defects, commonly a bitemporal hemianopia. The exact visual field defect depends on the precise pattern of spread of the tumour, and whether the chiasm is pre- or post-fixed. Rarely, tumours may also compress the hypothalamus, leading to abnormalities in behaviour, appetite, thirst and temperature regulation. Extremely large tumours may cause hydrocephalus by obstruction either of the foramina of Monro or the aqueduct of Sylvius, which connects the third and fourth ventricles. Invasion of local structures not only results in tissue destruction but also reduces the chance of surgical cure.

Hypopituitarism

Local tumour growth may cause hypopituitarism either by obstructing the flow of portal blood which contains the hypothalamic releasing hormones

Table 3.1 The effects of pituitary tumour invasion

Direction of spread	Site	Effects
Inferior/anterior	Sphenoid sinus	CSF leak
lateral	cavernous sinus	cranial nerve palsy carotid artery invasion
	temporal lobe	epilepsy
superior	diaphragm	headache
	optic chiasm	field defects
	hypothalamus	abnormalities of behaviour, temperature, thirst, appetite
	foramen of munro	hydrocephalus
	aqueduct of sylvius	hydrocephalus

and inhibitory hormones which act on the pituitary, or by the destruction of normal anterior pituitary tissue. Thus, for example, the interruption of access of the hypothalamic inhibitory factor dopamine to the anterior pituitary lactotrophs may lead to hypersecretion of prolactin.

Typically, compression leads to loss of anterior pituitary function in the following order: (1) growth hormone (GH); (2) luteinizing hormone (LH); (3) follicle-stimulating hormone (FSH); (4) thyroid-stimulating hormone (TSH); (5) corticotrophin (ACTH); and (6) prolactin (PRL) secretion, which is rarely reduced, but in contrast is quite often elevated.[4] Hormone secretion by the posterior pituitary is affected only very rarely and abnormalities suggest a primary problem of hypothalamic rather than pituitary origin. It should be stressed that any combination of defects can occur—particularly after pituitary surgery or radiotherapy of a tumour.

Although this chapter concentrates on pituitary disease in adults it is important to be aware that the age of onset of pituitary hormone deficiency determines its effect. GH deficiency may be unimportant in utero, but primary or secondary GH deficiency results in impaired growth velocity in early childhood.[5] GH deficiency in childhood is expressed as impaired growth; an affected child is typically plump, with immature facies and small hands, feet and genitalia. GH deficiency in adult life is more subtle and results in an increased body fat-to-lean body mass ratio and may also result in a generalized lack of energy.[5]

TSH deficiency in neonates is potentially more critical, as both growth and neuronal development are dependent on a normal thyroid status.[6] However, these problems are seen almost exclusively with primary thyroid disorders rather than with hypopituitarism. While growth retardation responds well to thyroid replacement, neuronal development may not if treatment is delayed. Fortunately, this problem does not occur with hypothyroidism occurring later in childhood, which results in symptoms and signs similar to those of adults, with the addition of growth retardation.

Thus, presentation may be with weight gain, decreased energy, sensitivity to the cold, constipation and dry skin.

Gonadotrophin deficiency in utero does not alter sexual differentiation, although it may be associated with maldescent of the testes. There are no signs attributable to gonadotroph damage in childhood until a delay in onset of puberty is noted. In adults, gonadotrophin deficiency presents with amenorrhoea, dyspareunia, and later breast atrophy in women, and loss of secondary sexual hair in men.

PRL deficiency is only apparent in the puerperium after delivery, when lactation does not occur.[7] ACTH deficiency presents with pallor, weakness, tiredness, nausea, vomiting and, in advanced cases, with postural hypotension.[8] However, severe Addisonian features are very uncommon as the renin–angiotensin–aldosterone system remains intact in these patients. Panhypopituitarism may precipitate sudden collapse and coma with hypothermia, hypotension and hypoglycaemia.[8]

Hormone hypersecretion

Twenty-three per cent of all pituitary tumours are endocrinologically inactive, although many of these may secrete the α subunit of the glycoprotein hormones LH, FSH or TSH, and their secretion may respond to luteinizing hormone-releasing hormone (LHRH) and to thyrotrophin-releasing hormone (TRH).[9,10] the functional pituitary adenomas are most commonly PRL secreting (55%), followed by GH secreting (27%), ACTH secreting (4%), and combined PRL and GH secreting (12%) adenomas; the remainder are gonadotrophin secreting (1–2%) and the rare TSH-secreting tumours. The mode of presentation of each is described.

Prolactinoma

Prolactinomas are the most common pituitary tumours. They are far more common in women, at a ratio of 20 : 1. They are rare during childhood, but can present with delayed puberty. In the adult female, presentation may be with a combination of galactorrhoea, oligomenorrhoea, luteal phase defect or occasionally, when periods persist, infertility. Infertility without amenorrhoea, may be due to anovulatory cycles or the direct inhibitory effect of PRL on luteal progesterone production.[11,12] Interestingly, and in contrast to other hypogonadal states, breast atrophy does not occur with hyperprolactinaemia although, paradoxically, galactorrhoea may not always be present.[13] The lack of galactorrhoea is more common with higher levels of PRL (associated with more severe hypogonadism) and may be because a permissive level of oestrogen is necessary for galactorrhoea to occur.[13] Men typically present with symptoms and signs of hypogonadism, with or without gynaecomastia, and only extremely rarely with galactorrhoea. Not

Table 3.2 Effects of Growth Hormone hypersecretion

System	Organ/structure	Complication
musculoskeletal	hands and feet	increased size, "spade" like
	face	coarse features, prognathism, frontal bossing
	joints	arthropathy, spondylitis,
	spine	kyphosis
	muscle	proximal myopathy,
	skin	thick and greasy, papillomata, lipomata, sweating
nervous	peripheral nerves	nerve entrapment, hypertrophic neuropathy
miscellaneous	visceromegaly	thyroid, kidney, liver, spleen
respiratory	upper respiratory tract	obstruction, sleep apnoea
	lung	increased capacity
	voice	deepening
metabolic	pancreas	diabetes mellitus
	calcium metabolism	hypercalcaemia hypercalcuria (renal stones)
cardiovascular	heart	cardiomyopathy
	vascular	hypertension, atheroma

infrequently, the diagnosis may be made by chance following other investigations, such as a skull X-ray after trauma.

GH-secreting adenoma

The prevalence of acromegaly is 30–50 per million of the population. Presentation before puberty, and hence before epiphyseal fusion has occurred, is rare and is the cause of pituitary gigantism. In the adult, the usual mode of presentation is with somatic changes such as malocclusion from the prognathic growth of the mandible, increased size of the hands and feet, or coarsening of the facial features. These signs are insidious, and a remarkably long time may pass before presentation. Other features of acromegaly which lead to its presentation include headache, sweating, carpal tunnel syndrome and diabetes mellitus. Visual field defects may be found in those who present late in the course of the disease.

GH hypersecretion may affect several body systems as shown in Table 3.2, and is associated with an increased risk of malignancy, particularly of colon and breast. Overall mortality is increased twofold in patients with active acromegaly, predominantly due to the cardiovascular complications.[14]

ACTH-secreting adenoma

These adenomas are rare. They are commoner in women (8 : 1), occur most frequently between the ages of 20 and 60 years and account for 70%

Table 3.3 Clinical features of Cushing's syndrome

System	Organ/structure	Complication
reproductive	pituitary	amenorrhea, impotence
	uterus/placenta	miscarriage, preterm labour
metabolic	pancreas	diabetes mellitus
	renal	hypokalaemic alkalosis
cardiovascular	heart	cardiomyopathy
	vascular	hypertension, atheroma
musculoskeletal	general	central obesity, peripheral wasting, buffalo hump,
	face	moon face, hirsutism, acne, plethoric,
	bone	osteoporosis
	muscle	proximal myopathy
	skin	bruising, thinning, striae
nervous	brain	psychiatric disorder
haematological	white cells	polymorphocytosis, lymphopenia, infections
	red cells	polycythaemia
miscellaneous		peptic ulceration impaired wound healing

of all cases of Cushing's syndrome. Oversecretion of ACTH increases the circulating level of cortisol resulting in Cushing's syndrome. The clinical features are shown in Table 3.3. Most patients present with the facial and truncal changes of Cushing's syndrome, and hypertension and diabetes mellitus are common. It is a severe disease with an untreated mortality of 50% at 5 years.[15]

TSH-secreting adenomas

These tumours are very rare. Presentation is with hyperthyroidism and inappropriate non-suppressed circulating levels of TSH. Although these tumours have been suggested to arise as a result of long-standing hypothyroidism, there is little evidence to support this, and when the association has been described the tumours regress with thyroxine treatment, and probably represent separate thyrotroph hyperplasia.[16]

Gonadotroph-secreting adenomas

Gonadotroph-secreting adenomas are increasingly recognized as a major component of the endocrinologically inactive group of pituitary tumours. Only rarely do they synthesize and release inappropriately high concentrations of gonadotrophin hormones. More often, they selectively release the α subunit of these hormones and the release of this subunit can be enhanced with both gonadotrophin-releasing hormone (GnRH) and TRH.[9,10] Therefore, these tumours would seem to have lost the ability to synthesize the β subunit, combine the two subunits or release the whole molecule.

Most patients present with symptoms of chiasmal compression rather than hormonal dysfunction. Gonadotrophin-secreting adenomas have been suggested to arise in patients with long-standing hypogonadism, but as these sella masses may regress with sex steroid replacement, they are likely to represent gonadotroph hyperplasia.[17] Furthermore, hypogonadal post-menopausal women do not have an increased incidence of these tumours.

Multiple endocrine neoplasia

Rarely, pituitary tumours occur in association with parathyroid adenoma, pancreatic tumour and adrenal cortical tumours in multiple endocrine neo-plasia (MEN) type 1.[18] Adrenal medulla tumours may occur with para-thyroid or thyroid medullary cell carcinoma in MEN 2 (1). Although, these divisions and the subdivisions of the type 2 syndrome usually define all cases of MEN, pituitary tumours may occur with phaeochromocytomas in overlap states. Pituitary tumours occurring in this condition should be managed in the same manner as those in non-MEN patients. In addition, annual screening for MEN (1) is recommended, and performed by clinical examination and the biochemical assessment of basal circulating calcium, calcitonin, PRL and GH levels, together with those of pancreatic polypeptide and glucagon levels after a test meal.

DIAGNOSIS

Biochemistry

Non-functioning adenoma

Elevated gonadotrophin levels (typically FSH) may be found in a small number of patients with non-functioning adenomas.[19] A higher proportion have an elevation in the circulating levels of α subunit.[19] These may be increased further during LHRH or TRH tests;[10] although this is of interest and of potential importance in the evaluation of the response to new therapies, it does not help in the management of most cases. The biochemical assessment needed in these patients is simply to identify hypopituitarism. In most cases this may be accomplished by taking a good history and the baseline measurement of 9:00 a.m. cortisol and thyroid function tests, with an LH and FSH, and either a testosterone or oestradiol. A Synacthen test may be required if the cortisol status is unclear, although this is not usually necessary as a preoperative procedure since the patient will have peri-operative steroid cover.

Table 3.4 The differential diagnosis of hyperprolactinaemia

Groups	Condition
physiological	pregnancy lactation stress excercise
pathological	hypothalamic disease: tumours, granuloma, stalk transection pituitary disease: prolactinoma, acromegaly, empty sella
dopamine antagonists	neuroleptics: chlorpromazine antiemetics: metoclopramide antihypertensives: reserpine
miscellaneous	chronic renal failure primary hypothyroidism polycystic ovary syndrome oestrogen treatment chest wall lesions

Prolactinoma

The upper limit of 'normal' of a basal circulating PRL varies depending on the nature of the assay used. Generally, levels of greater than 400 mU/I or 20 ng/ml are considered to be elevated. A single finding should be confirmed by repeated testing. In some patients, PRL levels may be elevated by stress. If a patient finds venesection to be particularly stressful, a cannula may be used and repeated measurements made over a 2 h period. The differential diagnosis of hyperprolactinaemia is long (see Table 3.4). A full history is vital and all non-pituitary causes of hyperprolactinaemia must be excluded before the diagnosis of a prolactinoma is considered. Many tests have been suggested to help in the definitive diagnosis of a prolactinoma. These include dynamic tests with a dopamine antagonist (metoclopramide 5–10 mg), TRH (200 μg) or even insulin-induced hypoglycaemia. It is true that these fail to increase circulating levels of PRL in about 90% of prolactinomas, unlike their effect in normal subjects.[20] However, they do not distinguish between a hypothalamic or pituitary aetiology of the hyperprolactinaemia. This is best achieved, once a non-pituitary cause of the hyperprolactinaemia has been excluded (Table 3.4), by imaging of the pituitary fossa, preferably with magnetic resonance imaging (MRI), which will differentiate between pituitary micro- and macroadenomas and hypothalamic lesions, such as a craniopharyngioma.

Generally, a macroadenoma associated with circulating PRL levels of at least 6000 mU/I is a genuine PRL-secreting tumour.[21] However, inter-mediate levels, between 4000 and 6000 mU/I, are in a grey area, and the differential diagnosis between a prolactinoma and an endocrinologically inactive tumour with stalk compression may only be possible after a trial of dopamine agonist therapy to assess possible reduction in tumour size. Usually, macroadenomas with prolactin levels below 4000 mU/I are due to disconnection of the pituitary lactotrophs from hypothalamic dopamine inhibition due to pressure from the non-secreting tumour.

In the absence of a macroadenoma, disconnection hyperprolactinaemia related to an intrasellar microadenoma is very unlikely, and raised PRL levels almost always represent a microprolactinoma. In the absence of a mass in the pituitary fossa, one can only conclude that the patient has either idiopathic hyperprolactinaemia, probably of hypothalamic origin, a microadenoma which is too small to be visualized or lactotroph hyperplasia.

Acromegaly

The biochemical diagnosis of acromegaly is based in the demonstration of a random GH of >10 mU/l (5.0 ng/ml), failure of suppression to <2.0 mU/I (1.0 ng/ml) following an oral glucose load of 75 g, and an elevated insulin-like growth factor 1 (IGF-1) level (corrected for age, and with normal nutrition, liver and renal function). Although it is of considerable interest that, unlike normal somatrophs, somatroph adenomas often release GH in response in TRH, and sometimes LHRH, but fail to respond to insulin-induced hypoglycaemia, these tests add little to the diagnosis or management of acromegaly. Neither do they identify those patients who are likely to have been cured after surgery. However, such tests may confirm cases of hypopituitarism (see above). In less than 1% of cases of acromegaly, hypothalamic (or ectopic) production of GHRH may be the cause of the GH hypersecretion. These cases may be detected by assay of the circulating levels of GHRH, which should be performed only in those cases of acromegaly in which no adenoma can be demonstrated in the pituitary fossa. Prolactin measurements should also be made in all cases of acromegaly in order to identify cases of mammo-somatotroph adenomas which co-secrete prolactin and growth hormone and which are often sensitive to treatment with Bromocriptine.

ACTH-secreting adenoma

The primary diagnosis of cortisol overproduction is best made by demonstration of raised 24 h excretion of urinary free cortisol, loss of diurnal rhythm of plasma (or salivary) cortisol and lack of overnight suppression of cortisol in response to a low dose (1 mg) of dexamethasone.[22] Further information may be gained from a full combined low-dose and high-dose dexamethasone suppression test, which in Cushing's disease but not adrenal adenoma will show inhibition of cortisol secretion during the high-dose (8 mg) dexamethasone stage of the test. CRH testing may be of value both in the differential diagnosis of Cushing's syndrome and in the follow-up of patients with treated Cushing's disease. A single intravenous bolus of

CRH-41 (100 μg) will evoke a normal or exaggerated response in Cushing's disease, and no response in the cases of ectopic ACTH or adrenal tumours. Other diagnostic tests such as loss of the cortisol response to insulin-induced hypoglycaemia or the metyrapone test are rarely of additional value. Adrenal adenomas are usually well seen on abdominal computed tomographic (CT) or MRI scans.

The presence of detectable ACTH levels implies ACTH dependence of cortisol secretion. Very high levels of ACTH, pigmentation and hypokalaemic alkalosis suggest ectopic secretion, most commonly from an oat cell carcinoma of the bronchus. Modest elevations of ACTH, with levels of cortisols which may be suppressed by high-dose dexamethasone, suggest Cushing's disease, confirmation of which may be gained by imaging of the pituitary fossa, preferably with MRI. Interpretation of the MRI scan should be by specialist radiologists together with the endocrinologist since not only may some ACTH secreting adenomas not be visible even after gadolinium enhancement, but non-secreting 'incidentalomas' may also be on high resolution scans and be misinterpreted as the source of ACTH. Indeed it may be impossible to be sure of the diagnosis even from apparently positive or negative radiology—and further advances in scanning technology may actually make diagnosis no more dependable.

Ectopic secretion of ACTH by tumours such as bronchial carcinoids may mimic Cushing's disease, and if this is suspected chest Xray and lung or abdominal scans may be indicated. When the diagnosis is uncertain, or the site of the adenoma is not clear from imaging of the pituitary fossa, petrosal sinus sampling before and after the administration of intravenous corticotrophin-releasing factor (CRH) may localize the tumour.[23] Petrosal sinus: peripheral blood ratios of ACTH of more than 2.0 in the basal state and more than 3.0 after CRH strongly suggest pituitary dependent rather than ectopic ACTH as the cause of the Cushing's syndrome. The relative levels of ACTH in left and right petrosal sinus samples may also help localisation of an 'invisible' adenoma in some cases.

TSH-secreting adenoma

Detectable circulating levels of TSH in the presence of hyperthyroidism suggest a TSH-secreting adenoma. The diagnosis may be confirmed by the concomitant detection of circulating α subunit (not usually necessary) and the presence of a mass on imaging of the pituitary fossa.

Imaging of the pituitary fossa (see Ch. 5)

A plain skull X-ray will detect a deformed pituitary fossa, bulging or ballooning of the fossa floor, destruction of the clinoids, calcification in a tumour and some of the changes of acromegaly. As air and metrizamide encephalography and angiography were superseded by CT scanning, so now CT has been superseded by MRI.[24] The only situation in which CT scanning is superior to MRI in the imaging of the pituitary fossa is in the assessment of bony invasion[25] and in the demonstration of calcification within tumours. The ability of MRI to differentiate between soft tissues in the assessment of spread of macroadenomas, and its superior ability to visualize microadenomas make it the imaging technique of choice in the pre-operative assessment of the pituitary fossa.[24,25] Its more widespread use is limited only by availability and price.

Petrosal sinus sampling

This has already been discussed under the diagnosis of Cushing's syndrome when neither CT nor MRI is able to visualize the tumour, or the question of the presence of an incidentaloma arises. In these cases bilateral simultaneous petrosal sinus sampling with or without CRF testing may be of use.[23]

Visual field assessment (see Ch. 4)

Goldman perimetry fields should be performed in all cases when the tumour extends into the suprasellar region. The sensitivity of the test is less than that of computer-assisted field assessments.[26] Nevertheless they provide a valuable adjunct in the repeated assessment of a macroadenoma. Hemi-field visually evoked responses (VERs) and changes in colour perception are also helpful in patients with chiasmal compression who are being assessed for response to medical treatment.

MANAGEMENT

Non-functioning adenomas

If there are no symptoms or signs due to pressure on the chiasm or other structures it is perfectly acceptable to follow patients with serial visual field estimations and MRI scans—initially every 3 months and then extending the period between scans up to 5 years when there is no evidence for any change in size of the tumour. If however there is evidence of visual field limitation or increase in size of the tumour, surgical decompression is necessary (see Chapter 6), usually in combination with post-operative radiotherapy (see Chapter 9). Although these tumours have a variety of functional receptors, no form of pharmacologically effective drug therapy is yet available.

Prolactinoma

The unique sensitivity of prolactinomas to dopamine agonist therapy makes these drugs the optimal primary treatment for both macroadenomas and microadenomas.[27] In some centres, surgery is performed as first-line treatment for microadenomas, although there is a significant recurrence rate post surgery and patients may be left with pituitary hormone deficiency. In view of the great number of patient years' experience with bromocriptine, this is the drug of first choice.

Bromocriptine should be introduced at low doses with food, and gradually increased to achieve optimum control. The first dose (1 mg) should be given with food at night; the dose may be increased after 2–3 days if a rapid response is required, or more gradually if the clinical situation allows. The final dose should be in the region of 5–15 mg/day in divided doses. When PRL suppression has been achieved the dose may be reduced to a level which maintains suppression of PRL levels.

After 2–3 years of treatment bromocriptine may be reduced and occasionally withdrawn if PRL levels remain within the normal range. Those who are unable to tolerate bromocriptine orally may find it more acceptable administered vaginally or could be tried on an alternative dopamine agonist (such as pergolide carbergoline or quinagolide) before resorting to alternative treatment in the form of surgery and radiotherapy. Even in patients presenting with visual defects due to chiasmal compression, the remarkable ability of dopamine agonists to shrink the majority of prolactinomas makes these drugs, rather than surgery or radiotherapy, the treatment of first choice.[27] It is important to monitor visual fields and tumour size (by imaging of the pituitary fossa) in a patient on treatment since some prolactinomas are refractory to dopamine agonist therapy. Thus, if no improvement is observed in the visual fields or VERs after 4 weeks of therapy surgery should be recommended. This should be followed immediately by radiotherapy in those who have persistent hyperprolactinaemia. Those who appear to be cured post surgery should be followed at regular intervals and if hyperprolactinaemia recurs, then surgery and/or radiotherapy will be needed.

In those patients with a microadenoma who desire to become pregnant, bromocriptine should be continued until a positive pregnancy test and then stopped. There is no evidence to suggest that bromocriptine is teratogenic. This risk of symptomatic tumour enlargement during pregnancy is of the order of 2–5.5% for treated microadenomas and up to 37% for macroadenomas.[28] These figures are drawn from the analysis of several studies, most carried out when the estimation of the size of a pituitary tumour was based on the size of the pituitary fossa. A more recent study assessed microprolactinoma size before and after pregnancy by CT scanning.[29] Tumour enlargement occurred in all patients, but was symptomatic in one only. In this patient, the tumour grew from 8.5 mm in diameter to 11 mm and caused headaches but no visual field defect. In the remainder—all with tumours of less than 5 mm—although enlargement occurred, none became macroadenomas and none was symptomatic. This small series, and our own clinical practice, suggests that those patients with tumours of less than 5 mm are unlikely to have problems during pregnancy; the remainder with larger microadenomas, or macroadenomas, may, and should be kept under regular observation with visual field assessments and imaging of the pituitary fossa with MRI in those with symptoms or signs of tumour enlargement. In these patients, bromocriptine is usually effective and does not adversely affect the outcome of pregnancy.[28] In patients whose prolactinomas are resistant to bromocriptine, delivery or termination of the pregnancy brings about resolution of the symptoms and signs. Alternatively, in early pregnancy, transsphenoidal surgery may be necessary.

Ovulation induction should not be encouraged in patients with prolactinomas which are resistant to bromocriptine. During pregnancy, these tumours may require transphenoidal decompression or premature delivery of the fetus. Rather, definitive treatment of the prolactinoma should be pursued before ovulation induction is contemplated.

Acromegaly

Some GH-seceting adenomas (particularly those that co-secrete prolactin) are sensitive to dopamine agonist therapy, and in those who respond (20%) with normalization of GH and IGF-1 levels this should be the management of choice.[30]

The place for the long-acting analogues of somatostatin in those resistant to dopamine agonists is not clear. The need for parenteral administration, the frequency of two to four injections a day, the occurrence of gallstones and the expense all limit the use of the compound octreotide. There are, however, new formulations both of an alternative analogue called Somatuline, given by injection every 1 to 2 weeks,[31] and a slow release preparation of octreotide (octreotide LAR) which are currently undergoing clinical trials. The Somatuline preparation has been shown to be able to normalize GH and IGF-1 levels in most cases. Despite these exciting new advances in medical therapy, for the present time surgery will remain the treatment of choice for those who fail to normalize GH levels with dopamine agonists, with radiotherapy given to those who are not cured by surgery alone.

In patients who are resistant to dopamine agonists, unsuitable for surgery or still have active acromegaly despite surgery and/or radiotherapy, the use of the long-acting analogues of somatostatin is unchallenged although side effects, particularly cholelithiasis, may limit their use. Biliary ultrasound must be performed both before and during treatment. The benefit of somatostatin analogues used before surgery is still uncertain and awaits further data, although a short trial of their use with large tumours may be indicated as even a small reduction in size may increase the chance of surgical cure.

Once GH levels are controlled, cosmetic surgery may be considered, as, unlike the soft tissue changes of acromegaly, those due to bone growth, such as prognathism, do not reverse.

ACTH-secreting adenoma

Initial therapy with metyrapone reverses the side effects of raised circulating cortisol levels on blood pressure, connective tissue and immune function, which used to result in significant morbidity and mortality following surgery.[32] The definitive management of Cushing's disease is pituitary surgery in most cases trans-sphenoidal selective adenectomy by an experienced surgeon.

In view of the considerable morbidity and mortality of the condition, those in whom surgery is unsuccessful undergo pituitary radiotherapy, bilateral adrenalectomy and steroid replacement. The medical alternatives to adrenalectomy include metyrapone, the most commonly used agent, which blocks 11β-hydroxylase; mitotane, which destroys adrenal tissue; and ketoconozole, which both inhibits steroid synthesis and the release of ACTH. The long-term value of these agents in pituitary-dependent Cushing's syndrome is limited as each is associated with side effects. Metyrapone causes virilism, mitotane hypercholesterolaemia and ketoconazole liver damage.

Another group of agents act centrally by enhancing the activity of endogenous inhibitors or antagonizing endogenous stimulators of ACTH release. The more commonly used agents are bromocriptine (dopamine agonist), cyproheptadine (a serotonin antagonist) and sodium valproate (GABA transaminase inhibitor). None is universally successful, although individual patients may respond to one or other. Bilateral adrenalectomy carries with it the risk of Nelson's syndrome in approximately 20% of patients, and prophylactic pituitary irradiation should be carried out in all patients in whom this operation is performed. Even this does not present Nelson's syndrome in all cases so that follow-up is vital.

The treatment modalities of surgery and radiotherapy are discussed in other chapters and will not be considered here.

Hypopituitarism

The incidence of hypopituitarism postoperatively depends predominantly on the size and nature of the tumour; for microadenomas the rate is in the region of 3–5%, while for macroadenomas the rate is up to 30%, following transsphenoidal surgery. Any combination of pituitary hormone deficiency may occur. Some patients with selective or panhypopituitarism preoperatively may recover function after the operation; this phenomenon may be explained by decompression of pituitary cells, or the removal of the block of access of trophic hypothalamic factors to the pituitary cells. If radiotherapy has been given, formal assessments of pituitary function should be performed at 12 and 24 months and then biannually thereafter, since radiotherapy-induced hypopituitarism occurs at variable intervals after therapy.

Postoperatively, the majority of patients should be given routine hydrocortisone replacement until 24 h prior to the assessment of their hypothalamic–pituitary–adrenal axis. Although the insulin stress test used to be the gold standard for testing the hypothalamic–pituitary axis, it is now quite clear that this potentially dangerous investigation is unnecessary in most cases and has no place in modern endocrine centres, except for research purposes or for the specific investigation of GH reserve.

At 2 weeks post surgery, pituitary function testing may be performed simply, safely and accurately with a Synacthen test for cortisol response, together with basal estimations of the thyroid and gonadal axes.[33] Earlier than 2 weeks post-operatively, the Synacthen test may be inaccurate, and if the pituitary–adrenal axis needs to be tested an intravenous insulin test may be necessary. If the baseline thyroid or gonadotrophin estimations are equivocal, then formal assessment with TRH and GnRH tests may be performed. However, these are rarely useful unless performed as part of a research protocol. If GH response is also to be tested, assessment may be performed either with an insulin tolerance test (GH should rise to greater than 20 mU/l with hypoglycaemia of <2 mmol/l), which will also test the hypothalamic–pituitary–adrenal axis, or using GHRH. However, the GH response to GHRH is disappointing and variable. The diagnosis of GH deficiency is of clear importance in childhood, but its possible importance in adults has been recognized only recently and may have important consequences for patient well-being and cardiovascular risk.

Assessment of the resolution of hypersecretory endocrine activity is carried out in the same manner as the preoperative diagnosis: a baseline estimation of PRL for a prolactinoma and GH response during an oral glucose tolerance test (OGTT) for acromegaly or alternatively a simple profile of GH levels every 1/2 h for 2 hours together with measurement of IGF1. Assessment of a successful response to transphenoidal adenectomy in Cushing's disease can be performed at an early stage by measurement of low or even unmeasurable plasma cortisol levels at 9.00 a.m. Other tests include estimation of normal 24 h urinary free cortisols or a return to normal suppression of cortisol secretion following low dose dexamethasone. It is important to emphasise that patients whose Cushing's was due to non-pituitary disease (adrenal tumours or ectopic ACTH) will have suppressed hypothalamic-pituitary-adrenal axes and will be hypoadrenal for varying periods after cure of their primary disease.

REPLACEMENT

Hypothyroidism and hypoadrenalism may be managed by replacement with thyroxine and hydrocortisone, respectively. In suspected combined deficiency states which may have been present for a long time, treatment should be initiated first for the hypoadrenalism. The dose of thyroxine replacement varies between 50 and 200 μg/day and thyroid replacement should be tailored to maintain circulating levels of thyroid hormones within the normal range, as TSH levels are unhelpful in pituitary dependent hypothyroidism. Hydrocortisone replacement varies from 15 mg to 30 mg per day in divided doses. In our experience the most satisfactory regimen is to mimic the normal diurnal rhythm of cortisol by giving most of the dose on awakening and the rest at mid-day (e.g. 15 mg and 5 mg on wakening and at mid-day respectively). The determinants of adequate steroid replacement are undefined, and biochemical indices such as 24 h multiple sampling for cortisol may not correlate with the subjective response of the patient. The dose of cortisol should be tailored to avoid the symptoms of hypoadrenalism. Overdosage on the other hand is often first suggested by weight gain. It is our practice to reduce the dose of cortisol to 15 mg per day in patients of average stature, and if this results in symptoms suggestive of hypoadrenalism to increase the dose until the symptoms disappear. There is increasing evidence that even small degrees of cortisol excess are deleterious to health and we strive to avoid this if possible. Patients on steroid replacement should wear a steroid alert bracelet or necklace, carry a steroid card and be aware of and understand the need for increased steroid replacement during illness.

In the case of hypogonadism the treatment is less simple. The great majority of hypogonadal patients should be replaced with exogenous sex steroids, not only to ensure normal sexual function but also to avoid osteoporosis. While this problem has been recognized for some time in hypogonadal women, it has only relatively recently been identified in men. The additional benefit in women is on cardiovascular mortality. Replacement in men has to be by injection either 2–4-weekly with Sustanon or at 4–6-monthly intervals with a testosterone implant. Although oral preparations are available they rarely achieve adequate plasma levels. Testosterone patches are now coming on to the market, initially as scrotal patches, but soon in the form of normal skin patches and these will undoubtedly prove a popular alternative. In women, replacement should be with cyclical oestrogens and progesterone, unless the patient has had a hysterectomy, when replacement may be with oestrogens alone. Some women may complain of a reduced libido and testosterone implants may be added.

In those patients who would like to have children, fertility may be restored by the use of exogenous gonadotrophins. In women this may be achieved with human menopausal gonadotrophin (hMG) with ultrasound follicle tracking to monitor follicle maturation and to time human chorionic gonadotrophin (hCG) administration at a follicle size of 17–20 mm. In men, hCG should be administered first in order to restore Leydig cell function, and when the circulating testosterone levels have reached the normal range of 10–30 mnol/l, then either hMG or FSH may be administered in addition. In either males or females who fail to respond, occult GH deficiency should be borne in mind and replacement may be of benefit. GH deficiency in children is corrected by the use of synthetic GH. In adults, the symptoms of mild hypoglycaemia with a lack of energy and drive seem to be typical of a GH deficiency state. These may be reversed by the administration of GH by intramuscular injections two to three times a week.

Diabetes insipidus may arise after surgical intervention. Postoperatively it may not be permanent and there may even be a phase of SIADH (syndrome of inappropriate ADH secretion): the investigation and management of this are described in chapter 8. Diabetes insipidus is managed with DDAVP given as a nasal spray at a dose of 5–20 μg once or twice a day. An oral preparation is also available but needs larger doses (200–800 μg/day) and often 3 rather than 2 doses per day. In some patients where tumour invasion of the hypothalamus damages their sense of thirst, these patients have to be managed with a fixed fluid intake and DDAVP and need careful monitoring and also counselling on how to manage when they leave hospital.

Finally GH replacement is now being assessed in many specialist centres. It is clear that GH replacement in GH deficient adults results in a redistribution of body mass from fat to lean body tissue and also in some patients appears to cause a marked increase in subjective well-being. There are some problems with fluid retention and some anxieties about the possible risk of increased incidence of tumours. Currently GH replacement should only be given in specialist centres where all treated patients are fully recorded on an appropriate database for objective assessment of response to therapy.

PITFALLS IN THE DIAGNOSIS OF A PITUITARY TUMOUR

Occasionally, lesions in the pituitary fossa may masquerade as pituitary tumours. With more accurate imaging, conditions such as carotid aneurysms, empty sellae or arachnoid cysts should be identified pre-operatively. Others, however, will continue to cause problems; these include tumours derived from primitive germ cells (germinomas, dermoids and teratomas), gliomas (optic nerve glioma, oligodendrogliomas, astrocytomas and microgliomas), meningiomas, craniopharyngiomas, metastic tumours, granulomas (sarcoid, tuberculosis, histiocytosis X), abscesses and lymphocytic hypophysitis (seen particularly in the puerperium). Such pathologies usually present with hypopituitarism, although occasionally hyperprolactinaemia may be present. Clues as to the nature of the lesion may be gained from the presence of calcification, hyperostosis, extensive bony destruction or diabetes insipidus. The overall clinical picture may suggest the correct diagnosis; for example, carcinoma with metastasis, sarcoidosis, histiocytosis X, tuberculosis, recent or concurrent meningitis.[34]

PITUITARY TUMOURS DURING PREGNANCY

The effect of pregnancy on prolactinoma size and the management of prolactinoma expansion have been discussed earlier in this chapter.

Pregnancy is rare in active acromegaly, primarily because menstruation is disturbed in the majority of cases.[35] Pregnancy does not affect and is not affected by acromegaly.[36] If symptoms suggestive of tumour expansion occur during pregnancy, then in the first trimester termination should be advised followed by surgery; in the second and third trimesters surgery is an option with radiotherapy given in the puerperium. Similarly, pregnancy is rare with

Cushing's disease. The fetus appears to be relatively protected from high maternal levels of cortisol and there is evidence for placental conversion of cortisol to corticosterone.[37] Fetal adrenal suppression may occur, reducing dihydroxyepiandrostenedione (DHEA) production and hence placental production of oestriol. The low production of DHEA by the fetal adrenal is a reflection of its relative insensitivity to ACTH and the limited amount of ACTH which crosses the placenta to the fetal circulation. However, the outcome of pregnancy is poor, with increased rates of preterm delivery. As before, the timing of diagnosis determines the management. During the first trimester, the poor outcome of pregnancy means that termination and the initiation of appropriate treatment should be advised; in the second trimester metyrapone has been used without any adverse effects,[38] and in the third pre-term delivery should be induced. Exogenous steroids for the maturation of the fetal lung are probably not required in this situation.

One rare complication of pregnancy is the exacerbation of mild or borderline diabetes insipidus. The placenta makes an aminopeptidase which metabolizes vasopressin. If there is an inadequate reserve of pituitary vasopressin, then the patient may become symptomatic and require treatment with intranasal DDAVP. In the hypopituitary patient, at the time of delivery, increased parenteral steroids should be given and the dosage reduced in the puerperium.

PROTOCOLS FOR TESTS OF HYPOTHALAMIC PITUITARY FUNCTION

Thyrotrophin function

Assessment of thyroid function can simply be performed by measurement of basal levels of thyroid hormone. It should be noted that plasma TSH levels may be difficult to interpret after pituitary surgery.

TRH test

This is rarely needed as an index of thyroid function since sensitive TSH assays became available. Non-fasting state. 200 μg TRH given i.v. at time 0. Serum for TSH ($\pm$ prolactin, and + GH in acromegaly) at 0, 20 and 60 min. TSH should rise more than 2 mU/l to greater than 3.5 mU/l.

Gonadotrophin function

Assessment of gonadotrophin function can simply be performed by measurement of basal levels of LH and FSH together with plasma testosterone in men and oestradiol in women.

GnRH test

This is rarely needed. It may be given at the same time as TRH and Synacthen (or insulin) tests. Non-fasting state. 100 μg GnRH given i.v. at time 0. Serum for LH and FSH at 0, 20 and 60 min. LH and FSH should both rise to levels which depend on pubertal state and individual laboratory assays.

Growth Hormone

(a) Diagnostic tests for acromegaly.

Glucose tolerance test

Fasting state. 75 g glucose given at time 0. Samples taken at -15, 0, 30, 60, 90 and 120 min for blood, glucose and GH. GH should suppress to less than 2 mU/l.

IGF-1

A useful measure of mean GH activity. Normal ranges vary between laboratories.

(b) Follow-up for acromegaly. There is no simply way to measure cure, and a simple profile of GH levels every 1/2 h for 2 h is usually sufficient. Mean GH of less than 2 mU/l suggests cure, as does normalization of IGF-1.
(c) Tests for inadequate GH secretion. The importance of assessing GH reserve and giving GH replacement to adults is currently under dispute. If GH reserve is to be investigated it can be done by the following methods.

Insulin tolerance test

This investigation is contraindicated in patients with ischaemic heart disease or epilepsy and is also only rarely given to patients above 65 years of age. A doctor must be present at all times and have readily available intravenous glucose and hydrocortisone. An ECG must be performed before the test and must be normal. Hypothyroidism must be excluded. The test itself should be performed fasting: insulin 0.15 U/kg i.v. in normal subjects but 0.3 U/kg in states of insulin resistance (e.g. Cushing's or acromegaly) or 0.1 U/kg if hypopituitarism or hypoadrenalism is suspected. Blood sugar, GH and cortisol are taken at 0, 30, 60, 90 and 120 min. Blood sugar should fall below 2.2 nmol/l and GH rise to more than 20 mU/l.

Glucagon test

This is rarely used. Fasting state. Glucagon 1 mg s.c. Blood sugar and GH at 0, 90, 120, 180, 210 and 240 min. GH should rise to more than 20 mU/l.

GHRH test

Currently only a research test. Fasting state. GHRH 100 μg and serum for GH at −15, 0, 15, 30, 60, 90 and 120 min. Responses are variable, but GH should rise to more than 12 mU/l.

Corticotrophin (ACTH)

(A) *Test for Cushing's syndrome*
     Screening tests:
(a) 3 collections of 24 h urine production for measurement of urinary free cortisol. Normal range is less than 350 nmol/24 h for men and less than 300 nmol/24 h for women.
(b) Overnight Dexamethasone suppression test. 1 mg Dexamethasone at 11 p.m. Normal plasma cortisol the following morning should be less than 100 nmol/l and Cushing's is virtually excluded if the level is less than 50 nmol/l.

Diagnostic tests:

(a) Circadian rhythm study: normal values 09.00 hrs greater than 170 nmol/l, midnight less than 100 nmol/l. Loss of normal rhythm occurs in Cushing's syndrome.
(b) Low dose Dexamethasone test. 0.5 mg 6 hourly for 48 h. At 48 h plasma cortisol should be less than 50 nmol/l and on the second day urinary free cortisol should be less than 70 nmol/l.

Differential diagnosis of Cushing's syndrome:

(a) High dose Dexamethasone suppression test. Dexamethasone 2 mg 6 hourly for 48 h. Pituitary dependent Cushing's syndrome usually responds with fall of both 09.00 hrs plasma cortisol and urinary free cortisol on day 2 by more than 50%. An alternative high dose test is a single 8 mg dose overnight with measurement of 09.00 cortisol the next morning.
(b) Plasma ACTH. This is unmeasurable in adrenal tumours, typically 10–100 ng/l in pituitary dependent disease and greater than 200 ng/l in ectopic ACTH secretion. Ectopic ACTH secretion from carcinoid tumours often overlaps the pituitary adenoma range.
(c) Corticotrophin releasing hormone test. 100 μg CRH-41 is given intra-

venously and blood taken for cortisol at -15, 0, 15, 30, 60 and 90 minutes. A normal response reaches more than 50% above basal levels and this is exaggerated in pituitary Cushing's and reduced or absent in adrenal and most ectopic ACTH disease.

(d) Petrosal sinus sampling. After bilateral catheterization of the petrosal sinuses 100 μg CRH-41 is given. Samples are collected from both sinuses and a peripheral vein for ACTH at -5, 0, 5, 10 and 15 minutes. Microadenomas show an exaggerated ACTH response which may be localized to one petrosal sinus sampling catheter. Pituitary dependent Cushing's is suggested by a petrosal sinus: peripheral blood ACTH ratio of greater than 2:1 in the basal state and greater than 3:1 after CRH injection.

(B) *Tests for inadequate ACTH/cortisol secretion.*

Short Synacthen test

This must not be done within 2 weeks of pituitary surgery since the response of the adrenal glands to an acute injection of ACTH is a reflection of the adrenal gland's secretory capacity which in turn is dependent upon the degree of ACTH stimulation over the previous 2 weeks. If adrenal reserve must be checked within 2 weeks of surgery, an intravenous insulin test should be performed. The Synacthen test does not, of course, measure GH secretory response. Non-fasting. Synacthen (Tetracoasactrin, CIBA) 250 μg i.m. Plasma cortisol at 0, 30 and 60 min. Plasma cortisol should reach 500 nmol/l with an increment of at least 200 nmol/l.

Insulin tolerance test

(Protocol described under Growth Hormone section). The test is only valid if blood sugar falls below 2.2 mmol/l. Plasma cortisol should increase by at least 200 nmol/l and reach levels of greater than 500 nmol/l.

Glucagon test

This is less reliable than the short Synacthen or insulin stress tests and is rarely performed because of the relatively high number of false negative responses in normal subjects. Procedure as under GH and interpretation as for response to insulin stress test.

(c) Test for adequate hydrocortisone replacement. There is currently considerable dispute as to the value of measuring plasma cortisol (hydrocortisone) levels after hydrocortisone replacement. It is the authors' view that the patient's subjective feelings of well-being and lack of objective signs of overdosing (cushingoid facies, weight gain etc.) are the best ways to regulate replacement doses which are often given in excessive amounts. In exceptional situations a cortisol day curve may be of help.

Hydrocortisone day curve

Fast overnight. Take basal sample before morning dose and samples 1/2-hourly for 2 h, then 2-hourly until evening dose. Ideally, plasma levels during the day should be maintained between 1200 nmol/l (peak) and 100 nmol/l (trough) during the day, although biological activity is more prolonged and smoother than the pharmacokinetic profile.

Vasopressin (posterior pituitary) function

In the absence of symptoms of polydipsia or polyuria there is no need to investigate posterior pituitary function. If inadequate vasopressin secretion is suspected a simultaneous early-morning plasma osmolality (should be between 280 and 295 mOsm/kg) and urine osmolality can be performed which should show a urine-to-plasma osmolality ratio of more than 2 : 1. A more definitive test is as follows.

Water deprivation test

Patients must have adequate thyroid and adrenal secretion or replacement. If the patient is on desmopressin this should be stopped at least 24 h before the test. The patient should be weighed before the test, which needs to be terminated if the patient loses more than 3% of body weight. No fluid or food is given for 8 h and plasma osmolality is taken at times 0, 4, 6 and 8 h. Urine volume is measured 2-hourly and samples taken for osmolality at 0, 4, 6 and 8 h. At 8 h the patient is given desmopressin 20 μg intranasally or i.m. and urine is collected and measured hourly and aliquots taken for osmolality. In central diabetes insipidus urine osmolality fails to rise to more than two times plasma levels and plasma osmolality increases above 295 mOsm/kg during the water deprivation test; urine does, however, concentrate after desmopressin.

REFERENCES

1. Faglia G, Ambrosi B. Hypothalamic and pituitary tumours: general principles. In: Grossman A (ed) Clinical endocrinology. Oxford: Blackwell 1992; pp. 113–122.
2. McCormick WF, Halmi NS. Absence of chromophobe adenomas from a large series of pituitary tumours. Arch Pathol 1971; 92: 231–238.
3. Burrow GN, Wortzman G, Rewcastle NB, Holgate RC, Kovacs K. Microadenomas of the pituitary and abnormal sellar tomograms in an unselected autopsy series. N Engl J Med 1981; 304: 156–158.

4. Nelson AT, Tucker HSG, Becker DP. Residual pituitary function following transsphenoidal resection of pituitary macroadenomas. J Neurosurg 1984; 61: 577–580.
5. Christiansen JS, Jorgensen JO, Pederson SA, Moller J, Jorgensen J, Skakkabaek NE. Effects of growth hormone on body composition in adults. Horm Res 1990; 33 (suppl 4): 61–64.
6. Boyages SC, Halpern J-P, Maberley GF et al. A comparative study of neurological and myxoedematous endemic cretinism in Western China. J Clin Endocrinol Metab 1988; 67: 1262–1271.
7. Kauppila A, Chatelain P, Kirkinen P, Kivinen S, Ruokonenen A. Isolated prolactin deficiency in a woman with puerperal alactogenesis. J Clin Endocrinol Metab 1987; 64: 309–312.
8. Stacpoole RW, Interlandi JW, Nicholoson WD, Rabin D. Isolated ACTH deficiency: a heterologous disorder. Critical review and report of four new cases. Medicine 1982; 61: 13–25.
9. White MC, Daniels M, Newland P et al. LH and FSH secretion and responses to GnRH and TRH in patients with clinically functionless pituitary adenomas. Clin Endocrinol 1990; 32: 681–688.
10. Snyder PJ. Gonadotroph cell adenomas of the pituitary. Endocr Rev 1985; 6: 552–563.
11. McNatty KP, Sawres RS, McNeilly AS. A possible role for prolactin in control of steroid secretion by the human graafian follicle. Nature 1974; 250: 653–655.
12. Demura R, Ono M, Demura H, Shizume K, Oouchi H. Prolactin directly inhibits basal as well as gonadotropin-stimulated secretion of progesterone and 17β-estradiol in the human ovary. J Clin Endocrinol Metab 1982; 54: 1246–1250.
13. Kleinberg DL, Noel GL, Frantz AG. Galactorrhoea: a study of 235 cases including 45 pituitary tumours. N Engl J Med 1977; 296: 589–600.
14. Wright AD, Hill DM, Lowy C, Fraser TR. Mortality in acromegaly. Q J Med 1970; 39: 1–16.
15. Krieger DT. Cushing's syndrome. Berlin: Springer 1989; 293–320.
16. Scheithauer BW, Kovacs K, Randall RV. Pituitary gland in hypothyroidism. Arch Pathol Lab Med 1985; 109: 499–505.
17. Snyder PJ. Gonadotroph cell pituitary adenomas. In: Mollitch ME (ed) Pituitary tumours: diagnosis and management. Philadelphia: Saunders 1987; 755–764.
18. Thakker RV, Ponder BAJ. Multiple endocrine neoplasia. Clin Endocrinol Metab 1988; 2: 1031–1068.
19. Kwekkeboom DJ, de Jong FH, Lamberts SWJ. Gonadotropin release by clinically non-functioning adenomas in vivo and in vitro: relation to sex and effects of TRH, GnRH and bromocriptine. J Clin Endocrinol Metab 1989; 68: 1111–1118.
20. Klijn JGM, Lamberts SWJ, DeJong FH, Birkenhager JC. The value of the thyrotropin-releasing hormone test in patients with prolactin-secreting pituitary tumours and suprasellar non-pituitary tumors. Fertil Steril 1981; 35: 155–161.
21. Bevan JS, Burke CW, Esiri MM, Adams CB. Misinterpretation of prolactin levels leading to management errors in patients with sella enlargement. Am J Med 1987; 82: 29–32.
22. Crapo L. Cushing's syndrome: a review of the diagnostic tests. Metabolism 1979; 28: 955–977.
23. Oldfield EH, Chrousos GP, Schulte HM et al. Preoperative lateralisation of ACTH-secreting pituitary microadenomas by bilateral and simultaneous inferior pertosal sinus sampling. N Engl J Med 1985; 312: 100–103.
24. Johnson MR, Hoare RD, Cox T et al. The evaluation of patients with a suspected pituitary microadenoma: computer tomography compared to magnetic resonance imaging. Clin Endocrinol 1992; 36: 335–338.
25. Stein AL, Levenick MN, Kletzky OA. Computer tomography versus magnetic resonance imaging for the evaluation of suspected pituitary adenomas. Obstet Gynecol 1989; 73: 996–999.
26. Melen O. Neuro-opthalmologic features of pituitary tumours. In: Mollitch ME (ed) Pituitary tumours: diagnosis and management. Philadelphia: Saunders 1987; 585–608.
27. Management of prolactinoma. Lancet 1990; 336: 332.
28. Mollitch ME. Pregnancy and the hyperprolactinaemic woman. N Engl J Med 1985; 312: 1364–1370.
29. Toffle RC, Webb SM, Tagatz GE et al. Pregnancy-induced changes in prolactinomas as assessed with computed tomography. J Reprod Med 1988; 33: 822–826.

30. Besser GM, Wass JAH, Thorner MO. Bromocriptine in the medical management of acromegaly. Adv Biochem Psychopharmacol 1980; 23: 191–198.
31. Johnson MR, Chowdrey HS, Thomas F, Grint C, Lightman SL. The pharmokinetics and efficacy of the long acting somatostatin analogue somatuline in acromegaly. Eur J Endocrinol 1994; 130: 229–234.
32. Child DF, Burke CW, Burley DM, Rees LH, Fraser TR. Drug control of Cushing's syndrome: combined aminoglutethamide and metyrapone therapy. Acta Endocrinol 1979; 82: 330–341.
33. Stewart PM, Corrie J, Seckl JR, Edwards CRW, Padfield PL. A rational approach for assessing the hypothalamo-pituitary adrenal axis. Lancet 1988; i: 1208–1210.
34. Post KD, McCormick PC, Bello JA. Differential diagnosis of pituitary tumors. In: Mollitch ME (ed) Pituitary tumours: diagnosis and management. Philadelphia: Saunders 1987; 609–646.
35. Jadresic A, Banks LM, Child DF et al. The acromegaly syndrome. Q J Med 1982; 202: 189–204.
36. Fisch RO, Prem KA, Feinberg SB, Gehrz RC. Acromegaly in a gravida and her infant. Obstet Gynecol 1974; 43: 861–866.
37. Mitchell BF, Seron-Ferre S, Hess DL, Jaffe RB. Cortisol production and metabolism in the late gestation rhesus monkey fetus. Endocrinology 1981; 108: 916–924.
38. Gormley MJJ, Hadden DR, Kennedy TL, Montgomery DAD, Murnaghan GA, Sheridan B. Cushing's syndrome in pregnancy: treatment with metyrapone. Clin Endocrinol 1982; 16: 283–293.

CHAPTER

4 | The visual manifestations of pituitary tumours

Ian McDonald

Approach to the patient with visual failure
Visual symptomatology
Findings on examination
References

An understanding of the way in which the visual system is affected by pituitary tumours is important for two reasons. First, a change in eyesight is a common mode of presentation when these tumours have extended beyond the confines of the pituitary fossa. Secondly, detection of asymptomatic involvement of the visual pathways can provide important evidence about the extent of pituitary tumours presenting in other ways. Since many patients are first seen with symptoms attributable to damage to the afferent visual system, I shall begin with a general account of the approach to the patient with visual failure and then discuss individual manifestations in more detail.

APPROACH TO THE PATIENT WITH VISUAL FAILURE

Two questions need to be answered when one sees a patient with visual failure: 'Where is the lesion?' and 'What is its pathological nature?' Clinical answers to the latter question come chiefly from the history, and to the former from the physical examination. The first step therefore is a detailed history of the mode of onset and the evolution of the visual symptoms.

Next, to provide evidence for localization (including whether just one or both eyes are affected) and to establish a baseline for monitoring progress and treatment, there must be a careful examination of the upper six cranial nerves. The particular relevance of this part of the assessment will become clear shortly. The standard neurological examination then follows in order to detect the spread of the pituitary tumour beyond the sella region.

The final stage of the neurological assessment involves selecting appropriate investigations to confirm the clinical localization and diagnosis, to provide more evidence about the pathological nature of the compressing lesion, and to plan treatment. Both X-ray computed tomography (CT) and magnetic resonance imaging (MRI) provide invaluable and complementary information. MRI, particularly with gadolinium-DTPA enhancement, is the method of choice for delineating the extent of the lesion and its relationship to important neural structures. CT scanning gives information about the involvement of bone and calcification, the latter not being revealed by MRI. Demonstration of calcification can be important in differential diagnosis, since it is very common in craniopharyngioma and is sometimes seen in meningioma, whereas its presence is exceptional (though not unknown) in pituitary tumours (Fig. 4.1). MRI should be the first investigation, and may be all that is needed pre-operatively. It is the method of choice for following patients post-operatively.

Examination of the visual evoked potential (VEP) with half field stimulation is sometimes helpful in localization and is particularly useful in monitoring progress in cases managed medically or when there is residual tumour after surgery.

VISUAL SYMPTOMATOLOGY

Symptoms due to optic nerve fibre damage

A common mode of presentation of pituitary tumours, especially chromophobe adenomas and prolactinomas (in males), is with visual loss. Acromegaly rarely presents with visual failure although visual loss may be found on testing in patients with macroadenomas. Patients frequently complain of a tendency to bump into objects on one or both sides, reflecting the frequency of unilateral or bilateral temporal field impairment. Patients may present with blurring of vision when central vision is affected early (as in direct compression of the intracranial optic nerve—especially likely with a post-fixed chiasm—or with scotomatous central field defects). Sometimes severe visual loss in one eye is discovered accidentally when the 'good' eye is covered, leading the patient to report sudden visual loss. That it has been in reality more gradual is usually suggested by finding optic atrophy which takes a month or more to develop.

It is noteworthy that patients do not complain that the abnormal field is *black*, but *blank*: they are unaware of visual stimuli. A positive complaint of

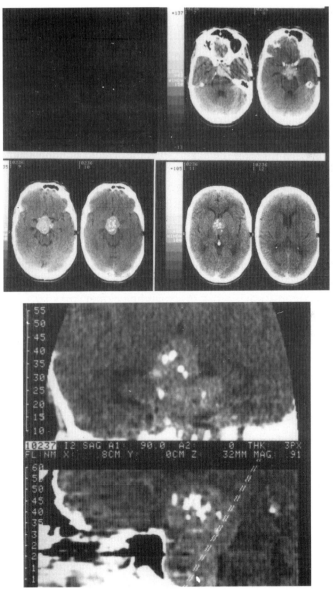

Fig. 4.1 (**a**) Axial CT (enhanced) of calcified prolactinoma. (**b**) Coronal and sagittal reconstruction of the same tumour.

blackness is usually due to retinal disease and not to lesions of the optic nerve fibres at any level.

Several unusual symptoms may be encountered as a consequence of bitemporal hemianopia. *Post-fixational blindness* occurs when there is a bitemporal defect which precisely splits the middle of the field.[1,2] In these circumstances, when a patient converges on a relatively close object, more distant objects fall in the blind hemifields behind the object of attention, and are therefore not seen. Symptomatically this is manifested, for example, by difficulty in cutting finger nails—focusing on the scissors results in disappearance of the nail—in sewing or occasionally in driving: focusing on the windscreen may result in the disappearance of traffic lights.

The presence of post-fixational blindness is readily demonstrated by confrontation. The patient is asked to focus on one of two objects held about 30 cm from the face. The other object is then slowly moved towards the examiner. When it enters the blind fields the patient no longer sees it.

A second group of symptoms derives from the phenomenon of *retinal slip*. The relationship between the fields contributed by each eye is normally preserved by a neurophysiological mechanism which depends on the stimulation of corresponding points in the homonymous hemifields. With a bitemporal field loss this is impossible, and the patient's visual perception depends on the function of two nasal fields which are not locked together. Slippage can thus occur. In the vertical plane the result is a tendency when reading to drop to the next lower line. Slippage in the horizontal plane can result in words running into each other or expanding: 'door' may become 'dor' or 'doooor'. One patient of mine, a bank clerk, was reprimanded for making errors of several orders of magnitude as zeros disappeared or were added to clients' balance sheets without his being aware of what was happening. An abnormal increase in separation of the nasal fields is sometimes reported as diplopia, and its cause must be distinguished from a defect in eye movement.

Positive visual symptoms

The symptoms described thus far are attributable to loss of function of the axons derived from the retinal ganglion cells. Occasionally patients experience spontaneous flashes of light which may be white, yellow or blue. Such symptoms are infrequently complained about, and their occurrence can more often be ascertained by direct questioning. They are probably due to the abnormal excitability which has been shown in central nerve fibres passing through a demyelinating lesion.[3] As will be described below, incomplete compressive lesions result in focal demyelination at the site of compression.

Neighbourhood symptoms

The commonest such symptom is *headache* which is presumably due to irritation of the dural lining of the pituitary fossa and the diaphragma sellae which are innervated by branches of the trigeminal nerve. It is present at some stage in about three-quarters of patients, especially in the early morning, but is not usually severe except in pituitary apoplexy when the abrupt onset of excruciating headache may simulate subarachnoid haemorrhage

(a)

(b)

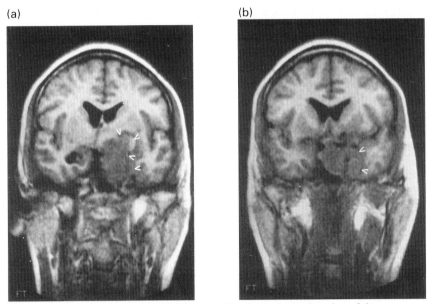

Fig. 4.2 Consecutive coronal MRI (T$_1$) scans showing extensive invasion of the cavernous sinus and compression of the medial temporal lobe (white arrowheads) by a prolactinoma. Note the void of the carotid artery surrounded by tumour in **b**.

from a ruptured aneurysm. The usual headache of pituitary tumour has no specific features; it is often felt behind the eyes, and may be referred to the vertex, especially in acromegaly.

Diplopia is usually due to paresis of one or more of the extraocular muscles and often signals lateral extension of the tumour to compress one or more of the ocular motor nerves in the cavernous sinus.

Rarely a patient may present with *temporal lobe epilepsy* when a giant pituitary adenoma spreads to involve this part of the brain (Fig. 4.2). Both major and minor seizures may occur. The latter include olfactory hallucinations, an intense experience of *déjà vu*, and a rising epigastric sensation. These features may appear in the aura preceding major attacks.

FINDINGS ON EXAMINATION

The most important part of the examination is that of the optic nerves and the eye.

Visual acuity

The visual acuity of each eye corrected with a pinhole (or by current refraction—remember that not all people keep their spectacles up to date) must be recorded for both reading and distance. The latter is particularly important, since many reading charts in current use are not standardized. The severity of impairment varies widely, and acuity is often normal in the early stages of chiasmal compression when only the peripheral fields are affected. When the field loss splits macular vision, the acuity is usually preserved, but the patient may read the letters only on the nasal side of the chart. A reduction of acuity in the absence of refractive error or incidental abnormalities in the media indicates that the field defect has crossed the midline.

Colour vision

Testing colour vision with each eye separately may provide invaluable evidence of even quite subtle pathological changes in the fibres of the anterior visual pathways. Impairment of colour vision is exceptional in retinal disease and a unilateral defect is almost always acquired; a bilateral defect is useful diagnostically if it is known (as it often is) that colour vision was previously normal.

Visual fields

The most useful single piece of evidence for localization of the site of compression is that provided by examination of the visual fields.[4] While the fields must always be recorded for future comparison, confrontation with a small red object can provide invaluable immediate evidence of hemianopias (bitemporal or homonymous) and scotomas.

In examining the fields by confrontation it is important to test both the peripheral and the central areas. The latter is best done with a small red object held halfway between the patient's and the examiner's eye and asking the patient to compare the quality of the colour when the object is moved quickly from a few degrees within the nasal field to a few degrees into the temporal field. Desaturation of the colour in the temporal field is an early sign of chiasmal compression.

Fields can be plotted with the Goldman or one of the automated perimeters (of which the Humphrey perimeter is currently one of the most popular) but in experienced hands the tangent screen is invaluable for revealing the details of field loss. Comparison of fields over time is facilitated by using the same symbols or colours on successive occasions—an obvious point which is surprisingly often forgotten.

Bitemporal hemianopia is one of the commonest findings with pituitary tumours, and indicates chiasmal compression (Fig. 4.3). The completeness of the hemianopia varies and depends on the size of the tumour and position of the chiasm. When the latter is markedly post-fixed, quite a large suprasellar extension of a tumour may not produce visual loss.

The field loss often begins unilaterally, when the intracranial optic nerve is compressed close to its junction with the chiasm. Early involvement of the decussating fibres from the nasal retina of the other eye (which subserves

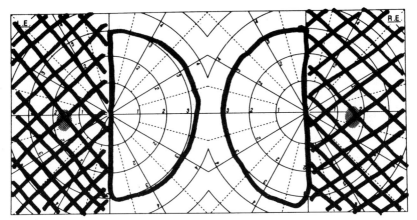

Fig. 4.3 Bitemporal hemianopia due to a pituitary tumour.

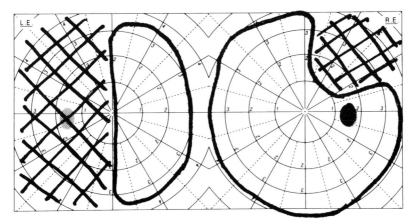

Fig. 4.4 Temporal field defect on the left with an upper junctional defect on the right due to a pituitary tumour.

the temporal field) is often signalled by a small contralateral upper temporal ('junctional') defect (Fig. 4.4). This pattern of field loss is attributable to the fact that the nasal fibres of the contralateral eye, after they have decussated, course anteriorly for a short distance into the optic nerve before looping back to join the fibres from the temporal retina to form the optic tract. Craniopharyngioma (which usually develops above the chiasm) often produces the converse pattern of field loss, with an inferior quadrantic defect on one side accompanying a complete temporal field loss on the other (Fig. 4.5).

More severe compression of chiasm and intracranial optic nerves results in the field defect's crossing the midline—a serious sign that requires prompt action.

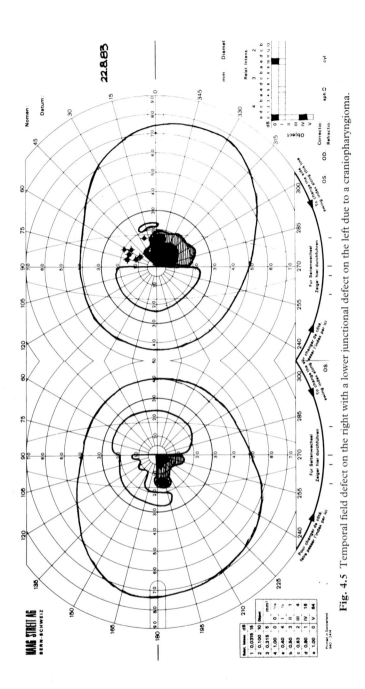

Fig. 4.5 Temporal field defect on the right with a lower junctional defect on the left due to a craniopharyngioma.

Another common pattern of visual loss when the chiasm is pre-fixed and the suprasellar extension of the tumour is more laterally rather than centrally placed is a homonymous hemianopia which is often incongruous, indicating compression of the optic tract.

Occasionally patients present with homonymous or bitemporal defects affecting the central few degrees of vision only, the latter pattern being attributable to involvement of the decussating fibres from the maculae at the posterior, inferior part of the chiasm.

Recovery following surgery

Decompression of the anterior visual pathways can result in a remarkably rapid and complete recovery of vision provided not too many of the optic nerve fibres have degenerated. The risk of irreversible damage is increased by both abrupt compression (as in pituitary apoplexy) and by prolonged compression, when severe optic atrophy reflects the severity of the nerve fibre loss.

In less severe cases the fields often open out within a day or two of decompression. This initial rapid phase of recovery is followed by more gradual improvement over weeks or months.[5]

A striking example of the speed with which the fields may improve—and of a number of the other features of involvement of the anterior visual pathways by pituitary tumour—is afforded by the following case.

A 36-year-old man presented with an 11-month history of difficulty in reading over his infant son's shoulder when the vision of the right eye was obstructed. On examination the corrected visual acuities were VR 6/5, VL 6/9. A scotomatous left temporal field defect and an incomplete upper right quandrantic defect detected by confrontation was confirmed by perimetry. There was temporal pallor of the optic discs but colour vision and the pupils were normal. A CT scan revealed a pituitary tumour with a large suprasellar extension. The patient had acted as a control subject for VEP recordings over a number of years; a striking change had taken place since the previous recording 32 months previously. The tumour was removed transcranially and proved to be a chromophobe adenoma. The patient had in advance agreed that I might examine him as soon as he awoke from the anaesthetic. This I was able to do approximately three hours from the time of decompression. The patient was drowsy, but co-operative. The field defects in both eyes were no longer detectable. Three days later formal perimetry with 1/1000 white object was normal. A VEP 10 days later showed a marked improvement and had returned to normal at four months.

This case highlights a number of questions about the mechanism of recovery of vision following decompression which have been investigated experimentally.[5] It is probable that the immediate recovery depends on the rever-

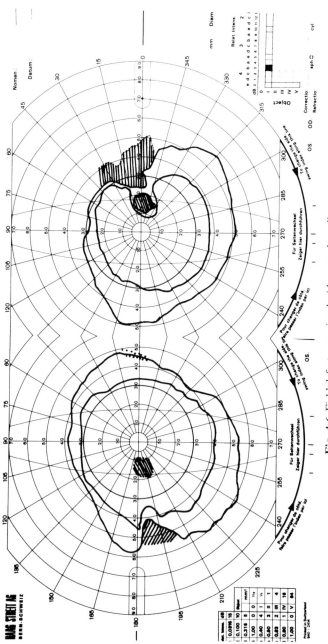

Fig. 4.6 Field defects associated with anomalous discs.

sal of ischaemic conduction block in demyelinated, remyelinated and morphologically intact nerve fibres. The slower phase probably depends on progressive remyelination and adaptive synaptic mechanisms to compensate for axonal loss.[7]

Unusual incomplete bitemporal or binasal field defects are occasionally found in asymptomatic individuals being examined for some other purpose, most often in the course of an assessment for spectacles. Such defects are often associated with anomalously shaped ('tilted') or hypoplastic optic discs (Fig. 4.6), and are of no pathological significance. If, however, there is any doubt about the cause of such defects, compression must be excluded by appropriate imaging.

Fundi

Fundal examination may reveal optic atrophy which indicates that compression is of long standing, or normal discs which indicate a potentially good prognosis for vision. The observation of an optociliary shunt vessel provides strong evidence against a pituitary tumour as the cause of visual loss, and in adults suggests the presence of a meningioma.

Papilloedema is excessively rare, and I have not seen it in several hundred personal cases examined over the past 25 years, though it has been seen when a giant pituitary adenoma blocked both foramina of Monro (M. Powell, personal communication). The importance of recognizing tilted discs has already been mentioned.

Pupils

A poor response to light with normal constriction on accommodation is to be expected with severe visual impairment. Of greater value in detecting more subtle damage of the optic nerves or chiasm is the demonstration of a relative afferent pupillary defect which is found with unilateral or asymmetrical involvement. The simplest way of demonstrating such a defect is as follows. The direct and consensual light reactions are examined on each side in the standard way. Pupillary constriction is observed. The direct reaction on one side is then re-tested and the light swung quickly to the other side. If the optic nerve on the second side is the more abnormal, the pupil will now dilate because the neural input to the superior colliculus from the ipsilateral side is less powerful (as a result of damage to the nerve fibres) than the contralateral consensual input. The test is best performed in low ambient illumination. It is important to exclude hippus as a cause of pupillary dilatation.

The orbit

The position of the eyes relative to each other and to the orbital rims should always be recorded. The presence of proptosis suggests a cause for the visual symptoms other than a pituitary tumour, most commonly a meningioma.

Other cranial nerves

Anosmia due to involvement of the olfactory tract is rarely seen with pituitary tumours; its presence suggests another cause for visual loss, most often subfrontal meningioma. Ocular palsies and involvement of the 5th nerve (of which a sensitive indicator is depression of the corneal reflex) provide presumptive evidence of the lateral extension of the tumour to compress the nerve in the cavernous sinus. This may occur acutely in pituitary apoplexy, but is usually gradual.

A striking finding with long-standing compression of the 3rd nerve is elevation of the eyelid on attempted adduction, due to abberant re-innervation of the *levator palpebrae superiorus* by regenerating fibres properly destined for the medial rectus. Since this sign occurring spontaneously is more commonly seen with meningioma involving the cavernous sinus and infraclinoid aneurysm of the carotid artery, its presence counts against a diagnosis of pituitary tumour.

FOLLOW-UP

A patient, who has had neurological manifestations of a pituitary tumour must be followed up indefinitely, since recurrence can occur even 25 years after surgery. Once the post-operative period (and radiotherapy, if it is required) is over and hormone replacement is stabilised, we follow patients in a joint clinic with endocrinological, neurological, neurosurgical, ophthalmological and radiotherapeutic staff.

Patients are usually seen after three and six months and then annually; later the follow up intervals are increased to 18 months to two years if the condition is stable. MRI is usually performed at alternate visits provided there has been no clinical change. It is essential, however, to instruct patients to contact their medical advisor if any deterioration in vision occurs.

If removal of the tumour has been incomplete or the patient is being managed medically, more frequent clinical and MRI assessments are required, the timing being determined by progress. Patients with prolactinoma may need to be followed initially at fortnightly or even weekly intervals. The frequency should be increased again during pregnancy.

REFERENCES

1. Nachtigäller H, Hoyt WF. Störungen des Seheindruckes bei bitemporaler Hemianopsie und Verschiebung der Sehachsen. Klin Monatsbl Augenheilk 1970; 156: 821–836.
2. Kirkham TH. The ocular symptomatology of pituitary tumours. Proc R Soc Med 1972; 65: 517–518.
3. Smith KJ, McDonald WI. Spontaneous and evoked electrical discharges from a central demyelinating lesion. J Neurol Sci 1982; 55: 39–47.
4. Glaser JS. Neuro-ophthalmology, 2nd edn. Philadelphia: Lippincott, 1990.
5. Kayan A, Earl CJ. Compressive lesions of the optic nerves and chiasm: pattern of recovery of vision following surgical treatment. Brain 1975; 98: 13–28.

6. Clifford-Jones RE, McDonald WI, Landon DN. Chronic optic nerve compression: an experimental study. Brain 1985; 108: 241–262.
7. Darian-Smith C, Gilbert CD. Axonal sprouting accompanies reorganisation in adult cat striate cortex. Nature 1994; 368: 737–740.

Imaging of the pituitary

Margaret Hall-Craggs,
W. K. Kling Chong,
Brian Kendall

INTRODUCTION

In recent years magnetic resonance (MR) has largely replaced computed tomography (CT) as the elective technique of choice for the cross-sectional imaging of the pituitary and parasellar region and there are a number of reasons for this. With few exceptions MR has been shown to be at least as good as CT, and in many situations superior, for the imaging of the pituitary and parasellar structures and associated diseases. As with all structures surrounded by bone, the pituitary is susceptible to bone-induced artifact on CT scans. In contrast, as cortical bone does not emit on MRI signal, images are free from the degree of bone-induced artifact suffered by CT. For adequate spatial resolution of the pituitary and associated pathology, thin slices are required. In order to generate sufficient signal-to-noise, this requires relatively high doses of ionizing radiation when using CT. MR does not use ionizing radiation (radio frequency radiation is used in the presence of a strong magnetic field). This is a particular consideration when imaging children and when repeated examinations are likely to be necessary.[1] Further advantages of MR include its capacity to image in any plane, thus obviating lengthy image processing times necessary for the reconstruction of CT scans. Three-dimensional data sets can also be acquired in reasonable imaging times and these can then be used for volume measurements and further image analysis.

There are some relative disadvantages of MR as compared to CT. MR is comparatively insensitive to the presence of calcification which can be a useful diagnostic aid. There are some absolute contraindications to MR scanning such as the presence of a cardiac pacemaker, an intracranial vascular clip or orbital metallic foreign body and these patients can only be scanned with CT.

MR SCANNING TECHNIQUES

The purpose of an MR scan of the pituitary is to show anatomy clearly and to generate contrast between normal and pathological structures. There are a variety of imaging options, with a choice between sequences (for example spin-echo or gradient echo, 3D or 2D). We use the following scan protocol. The brain is first surveyed using a T2-weighted spin-echo sequence in the transverse plane. Images of the pituitary itself with high spatial and contrast resolution are then acquired using thin slice T1-weighted spin-echo sequences before and after the administration of gadolinium-DTPA. Images are acquired in a coronal plane before and then in the coronal and sagittal planes after contrast enhancement. If the clinical problem is thought to relate to the posterior pituitary (for example in diabetes insipidus) the pre-enhancement scans are acquired in the sagittal plane. Gadolinium-DTPA is a rare earth chelate which behaves in a manner analogous to the iodinated contrast agents used in CT scanning. It causes shortening of the T1 relaxation time, hence tissue into which it crosses increases in signal intensity (i.e. becomes brighter) on T1-weighted images.

Occasionally it is useful to supplement these images with an MR angiogram to show the major blood vessels and vascular abnormalities such as aneurysm formation. This is a non-invasive technique which does not require the use of contrast agents. Flowing blood is seen as high signal against a background of low signal stationary tissue.

CT SCANNING TECHNIQUE

A plain CT through the sella and suprasellar regions using 5 mm sections is performed as a preliminary measure in all cases. This is to show any large masses and also any abnormal pre-contrast density. The normal size pituitary including those containing microadenomas are best examined by direct coronal imaging extending through the sellar region with the neck extended, using a scanning plane designed from the scout view image to avoid artifact from dental amalgam. If it proves impossible to achieve a satisfactory coronal position, thin axial slices (1.5–2 mm) are obtained at 1 mm intervals with the head extended about 10 degrees so as to place the petrous bones below the plane of the sella and thus avoid low-density artifacts generated from them passing through the pituitary gland. These images are reformatted in multiple planes as indicated for the elucidation of supra or peri-sellar extension of pituitary masses. The thin section images are made after bolus injection of intravenous contrast medium.

The nature of bone-induced artifacts will be evident on the original sections but they may simulate microadenoma on the reformatted images. Even with modern CT machines, a noise range of up to 10 Hounsfield units is to be expected in the region of the pituitary gland and this statistical electronic noise may simulate small tumours. In the absence of cooperative evidence, the constancy of such artifact can be confirmed by the routine use of dynamic scanning.

The density of the normal pituitary tissue is similar to that of normal brain; it lacks a blood–brain barrier (BBB) and enhances to a density similar to adjacent blood vessels after a bolus of intravenous contrast medium. With dynamic CT (Fig. 5.6) the posterior pituitary and pituitary stalk, which have a direct arterial blood supply enhance rapidly; the anterior pituitary, which is supplied by the portal venous system descending through the pituitary stalk, enhances more slowly and is less intense on early sections. The intensity of the anterior pituitary increases as the portal blood supply progressively opacifies during the minute following the injection and it eventually becomes denser than the posterior pituitary due to extravasation through the absent BBB. At this stage the less dense posterior pituitary can be shown with its convex anterior border impressing the posterior margin of the densely enhancing anterior pituitary. Colloid cysts remain unopacified and are less dense than normal tissue.

NORMAL ANATOMY AND APPEARANCES OF THE PITUITARY AND PARASELLAR REGION

The anatomy of the pituitary and the parasellar region is shown in the annotated Figure 5.1. (see chapter 6, Surgical chapter). The posterior border of the pituitary is formed by the dorsum sella. Laterally lie the cavernous sinuses through which the carotid siphon and the third, fourth and fifth cranial nerves pass. The anterior border is formed by the anterior wall of the sella and inferiorly lies the sphenoid bone, which is aerated to varying degrees.

The pituitary stalk or infundibulum lies in the midline and is about 2.5 mm in diameter, extending from the floor of the third ventricle and sloping forwards as it passes through the diaphragma sella to join the pituitary at

(a)

(b)

(c)

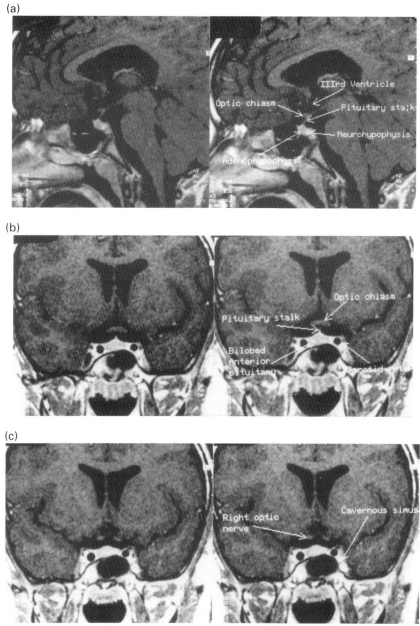

Fig. 5.1 Anatomy of normal pituitary. T1-weighted MRI. Sagittal (**a**) and coronal scans (**b**, at the level of the optic chiasm and **c**, at the level of the optic nerve). On the sagittal image, the signal from the posterior lobe of the pituitary is seen to be higher than the anterior lobe. In this peripubertal adolescent boy the gland is plump, with a convex upper margin.

the junction of the anterior and posterior lobes. Although usually a vertical structure in the coronal plane it can deviate slightly to the left or right by a few degrees in normal cases. The optic chiasma, which also lies obliquely, is situated at the anteroinferior extremity of the third ventricle, immediately anterior to the pituitary stalk.

On MR the pituitary can be clearly seen to consist of two lobes: the anterior and posterior. The anterior lobe has two lateral lobes, best seen on the coronal view, and occupies about four-fifths of the glandular substance. It is of relatively homogeneous intermediate signal intensity on T1-weighted images and is of a higher signal intensity on T2-weighted images.

The posterior pituitary is much smaller than the anterior portion of the gland and shows high signal intensity on T1-weighted images in over 90% of normal individuals. The substance responsible for the signal hyperintensity has not yet been identified conclusively. Proposed sources include lipid in pituicytes, a paramagnetic effect of phospholipids, neurosecretory granules in the posterior lobe, fat in the sella or fat in the marrow of the dorsum sella. However, fat or lipid have been excluded as the cause of the hyperintensity as experiments have shown that there is no chemical shift[2-5] and that in the majority of cases the high signal is not reduced by fat suppression.[6]

When gadolinium is given there is an orderly sequence of enhancement of the pituitary gland.[7-9] Within the first few seconds the infundibulum and the posterior pituitary enhance. Following this there is centrifugal enhancement of the anterior pituitary. The signal intensity of the pituitary becomes homogeneous after about 90s and is then followed by slow washout of contrast, this being slightly faster from the posterior than the anterior lobe. The course of pituitary enhancement mirrors the vascularization of the gland with an arterial supply to the posterior lobe and a portal venous supply to the anterior lobe. The cavernous sinuses enhance early and the non-enhancing III and V cranial nerves can then be seen within the venous sinus.

The appearances of the pituitary vary considerably with age. In the neonate the gland is rounder and brighter than in children over 2 months old.[10] Convexity of the upper border is seen in two-thirds of neonates and the signal is higher in the pituitary than the brain stem on T1-weighted images. After 2 months, the gland becomes flatter and isointense with brain and this appearance is maintained throughout childhood until puberty. In the first year of life, the anterior and posterior lobes can only be distinguished from each other in 60–70% of children[10] and so inability to visualize the posterior lobe is a frequent occurrence and should not be interpreted as a sign of neurohypophyseal insufficiency in the very young.

During puberty, the pituitary appears to undergo physiological hypertrophy. The gland becomes larger and more rounded and this effect is more pronounced in girls than boys (Fig. 5.1).[11,12] A convex upper border is seen in over 50% of teenage girls. With the exception of the first year of life and during puberty, the pituitary undergoes linear growth throughout

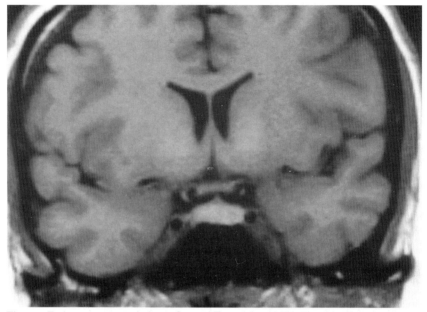

Fig. 5.2 Early post-partum pituitary. Coronal T1-weighted MRI. Five days following delivery of twins, this patient's pituitary is relatively large, with a convex superior margin. The gland measured 11 mm in depth, which is within the normal range in the early post-partum period. The signal intensity of the anterior pituitary is higher on T1 imaging than in the 'non-pregnant' gland.

childhood.[13] In adults of 21–40 years the mean height of the gland is just under 5 mm in men and 6 mm in women.[13] During middle age the pituitary begins to reduce in size and is significantly smaller than in young adults.[13,14]

During pregnancy the pituitary has been shown to increase in size in a linear fashion.[15] The height of the gland never exceeds 10 mm during pregnancy but is at its largest (up to 12 mm) in the immediate post-partum period (Fig. 5.2). Following the first week post partum, it rapidly returns to normal size irrespective of whether the mother breast feeds or not.

PITUITARY PATHOLOGY

Congenital variations and abnormalities

The pituitary gland traverses the diaphragma sellae through an aperture which varies in size in different individuals.[16] The arachnoid membrane accompanies the pituitary stalk through the diaphragm, and when the aperture is wide herniation of arachnoid may carry the chiasmatic cistern into the sella, which is correspondingly increased in volume to accommodate the cerebrospinal fluid (CSF) in addition to the pituitary gland. Such intra-sellar extension of the chiasmatic cistern has been shown in 54% of autopsies

(a)

(b)

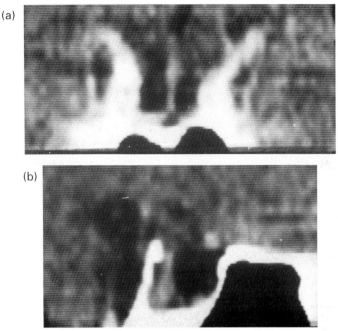

Fig. 5.3 Empty sella. Reformatted coronal (**a**) and sagittal (**b**) CT scan. The chiasmatic cistern extends deeply into the enlarged sella turcica outlining the pituitary stalk. A small amount of pituitary substance is present posteriorly in the sella.

and individual differences in the volume of intrasellar CSF has been shown to be the main factor responsible for the large normal variation in sellar size and configuration. In extreme cases, the pituitary gland is confined to the lower part of the sella, forming a thin rim along the floor and posterior wall (Fig. 5.3). This condition to which the misnomer 'empty sella' has been applied is usually an insignificant anatomical variant discovered incidentally when the skull is X-rayed for unrelated miscellaneous reasons. It may be an accompaniment of benign intracranial hypertension, and the relatively thin walls of the affected sella may occasionally be perforated and be the site of CSF leakage, causing rhinorrhea. The diagnosis of intrasellar arachnoid herniation is best confirmed when necessary by magnetic resonance imaging (MRI), which shows the fluid reflecting signal identical to that of the CSF elsewhere in the ventricles and subarachnoid spaces. The pituitary stalk extends through the sella to the pituitary substance lining the floor and posterior wall; it also shows the relationship of the structures within the chiasmatic cistern to the arachnoid herniation.

'Empty sella' may also be acquired following regression of a pituitary tumour due to surgery, radiation or hormone suppression therapy, or it may follow spontaneous infarction or haemorrhage into the pituitary tumour or infarction of normal gland substance (Fig. 5.4). In cases in which there has

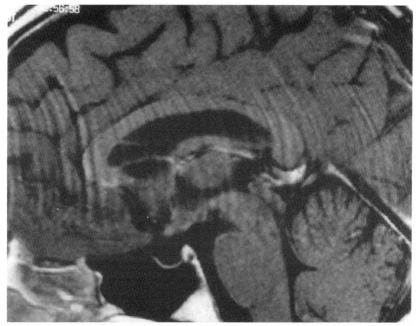

Fig. 5.4 Empty sella secondary to aseptic meningitis. Sagittal T1-weighted MRI. The sella, which is of normal size, contains only CSF. The pituitary stalk is atrophic and neither the anterior nor posterior portions of the gland are visible.

been regression of a tumour or an inflammatory process in which adhesions to the floor of the third ventricle—including the optic chiasm—may have formed, these structures may be drawn down into the sella. The altered anatomy is generally evident on MRI and the potential hazards of inappropriate transsphenoidal surgery thereby avoided.

The pituitary gland may be aplastic, hypoplastic or ectopic. In hypoplasia of the pituitary,[17] which may be associated with clinical and biochemical evidence of anterior pituitary hormone deficiency, the sella is small, but the infundibulum and pituitary stalk appear normal. The chiasmatic cistern may extend into the small sella.

Disruption of the infundibulum can sometimes be related to trauma in the perinatal period, and is more common in children delivered by the breach (Fig. 5.5). It interrupts the hypophyseal portal system, which impairs pituitary growth and function due to the lack of the releasing·factors produced in the hypothalamus. The anterior pituitary gland and the pituitary fossa are small, and the bright T1 signal of the neurohypophysis is absent from the usual site. It is commonly replaced by a T1 high signal nodule at the base of the infundibulum, which is developed in response to continued axonal transmission of posterior pituitary hormone and accounts for the absence of diabetes insipidus in such cases.[18]

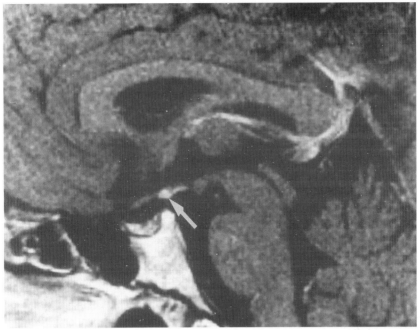

Fig. 5.5 Traumatic transection of the pituitary stalk. Sagittal T1-weighted MRI. The pituitary stalk is not visible. A high signal nodule (arrowed), probably due to accumulation of neurosecretory granules, is seen immediately proximal to the level of the stalk amputation.

Ectopic pituitary tissue

Pituitary tissue may develop anywhere along the route of the craniopharyngeal canal, usually represented by a few accessory cells. Rarely, a hypoplastic gland in a small pituitary fossa is associated with a large ectopic mass of anterior pituitary tissue.

Sphenoidal cephalocele

The craniopharyngeal canal normally closes at 50 days gestation. Continued patency of the canal is occasionally associated with Rathke cleft elements, or with a meningocele or encephalocele. The precise aetiology of the associated bony latter condition is uncertain, and the defect may include the posterior ethmoids, anterior wall and floor of the sella turcica as well as the region of the craniopharyngeal canal.[19] Craniofacial deformities are a constant accompaniment and should alert the clinician to the possibility of a transsphenoidal cephalocele in patients presenting with endocrine defects or a nasopharyngeal mass. Hypertelorism is constant and palatine and medial nasal fissures may be present as well as optic malformations, which include unilateral coloboma and hypoplasia of the eye, orbit, optic nerve or chiasm as well as retinal defects. The most typical presentation is with breathing difficulties or alteration of the voice associated with a nasopharyngeal obstruction.

The cephaloceles are best demonstrated by coronal and sagittal MRI. They contain the inferior part of the third ventricle with the infundibulum and hypophysis. The optic chiasm and first segments of the anterior cerebral arteries are usually deviated into the cephalocele, though the distorted anatomy may cause difficulty with precise delineation of the former. The bone defect is well shown by high-resolution thin-section CT. It involves the centre of the sellar floor, and typically extends anteriorly to involve the anterior wall of the sella, the presphenoid and sometimes the posterior ethmoid region; the dorsum sella is always normal.

Kallman's syndrome

This syndrome is characterized by a combination of anosmia or hyposmia with hypogonadotrophic hypogonadism. The combination has been explained by recent immunohistochemical studies.[20] At about 41 days of fetal life, the olfactory placode in the nasal fossa produces fibres and cells which migrate to lie beneath the telancephalic ventricles and form the olfactory nerves. The nerve fibres grow into the brain and induce the development of diverticuli from the telancephalic ventricles. The diverticuli close off to form the olfactory ventricles, which later are filled in to produce solid olfactory bulbs. Later, the cartilaginous cribriform plate forms below the bulb around the bundles of the olfactory nerves. Cellular migration also occurs from the medial part of the olfactory placode to reach the hypothalamic region and septum pellucidum, forming the medial septal nuclei, and specifically cells producing gonadotropin hormone-releasing hormones.

In Kallman's syndrome the olfactory axons fail to reach the forebrain or to induce the neuronal migration, resulting in the combination of olfactory hypogenesis or agenesis and absence of the gonadotropin hormone-releasing cells. High-resolution MRI in the coronal plane reveals hypoplasia of the olfactory sulci and olfactory bulbs. In some cases, abnormal soft tissue is shown in the region of the olfactory bulbs consistent with disorganized ectopic migrating neurones.

The condition is rare, with a frequency of 1 in 10 000 males and 1 in 50 000 females. It is most commonly transmitted in an X-linked recessive manner, but may be inherited as an autosomal recessive, and a dominant form has also been described. These forms may be distinguished by associated conditions determined by deletion of contiguous genes.

Tumours

Adenomas

Adenomas constitute the largest group of pituitary tumours and are classified by size into microadenomas (< 10 mm) and macroadenomas (> 10 mm)

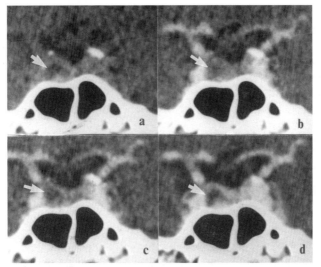

Fig. 5.6 Dynamically enhanced CT scan of pituitary adenoma. Coronal CT sections. The right-sided pituitary microadenoma becomes increasingly conspicuous as a region of relative low density (arrowed) during the dynamically enhanced scan.

(Fig. 5.6). In general microadenomas present because they are endocrinologically functional whereas non-functional macroadenomas present due to their size and subsequent compressive or invasive effects and this is reflected in their imaging appearances.

The majority of microadenomas are relatively well defined and are hypointense as compared with normal gland on T1-weighted images (Fig. 5.7). Less commonly they may be either hyperintense due to small cystic areas of haemorrhage within the mass (Fig. 5.8) or isointense. Depending on their size and situation within the gland they may cause some increased convexity of the upper border of the pituitary and deviation of the pituitary stalk. Microadenomas enhance less quickly and to a lesser extent than normal anterior pituitary tissue,[7] hence remain relatively hypointense and contrast between the gland and tumour is maximal early following enhancement (in the first 2–4 min). Occasionally adenomas may be predominantly cystic (Fig. 5.10) and rarely they may be more aggressive and destructive, simulating meningioma or secondary deposit (Fig. 5.9).

Macroadenomas undergo cystic degeneration and haemorrhage more commonly than microadenomas and therefore have more variable appearances. They may have signal characteristics similar to microadenomas and be homogeneous and relatively hypointense to the normal gland. Many, however, are heterogeneous, with regions of the cystic change appearing as lower intensity than solid tumour on T1-weighted images. Macroadenomas most commonly enhance with gadolinium and to a greater extent than the brain and this feature is helpful in demonstrating the full extent of the

(a)

(b)

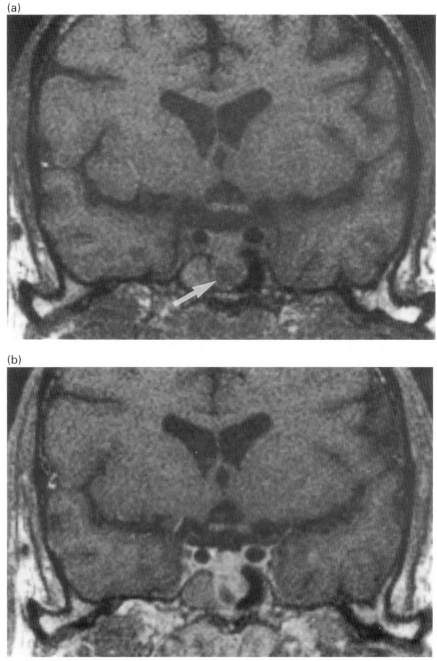

Fig. 5.7 Hypointense infrasellar adenoma. Coronal T1-weighted MRI before (**a**) and after (**b**) contrast. The floor of the sella is eroded and there is a hypointense mass (arrowed) within the sphenoid. There is no suprasellar or intracavernous extension of the mass. Following contrast the mass shows partial enhancement with relatively little enhancement centrally.

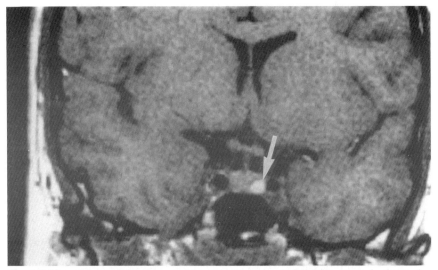

Fig. 5.8 Hyperintense microadenoma. Coronal T1-weighted MRI. A 6 mm prolactinoma is situated in the left lobe of the pituitary (arrowed). The high signal within the tumour before enhancement is probably due to haemorrhage.

tumour (Figs 5.11 and 5.12). The multiplanar imaging capacity of MR is very helpful for showing the full anatomic extent of macroadenomas and for pre-surgical planning. Suprasellar tumour extension and its relationship to the optic chiasm and hypothalamus and infrasellar tumour extension into the sphenoid can be clearly visualized on sagittal and coronal images. Normal pituitary tissue may be seen compressed in the sella or, with large tumours, it may not be visualized at all. Detailed bone structure is not shown as well by MR as CT and bone destruction cannot be differentiated from bone expansion and thinning.

The cavernous sinus may be infiltrated by both micro-and macroadenomas. MR is relatively poor for identifying cavernous sinus involvement by tumour, with a sensitivity of just over 50%.[21] Tumour involvement can vary from displacement of the medial wall of the sinus, through macroscopic infiltration of the dura to extensive invasion, with or without encasement of the carotid arteries (Fig. 5.12). The relationship between the pituitary and cavernous sinuses is most easily seen in the coronal plane and the most useful criteria for identifying cavernous sinus invasion on MR are asymmetric signal intensity of the invaded sinus and the presence of carotid artery encasement.[21] The major reason why MR is insensitive to cavernous sinus involvement is that the medial dural reflection (pituitary capsule) cannot be identified by MR and hence early dural infiltration cannot be distinguished from displacement.

Sudden expansion of the pituitary due to haemorrhage or infarction of a pituitary adenoma can produce the clinical syndrome of pituitary apoplexy.

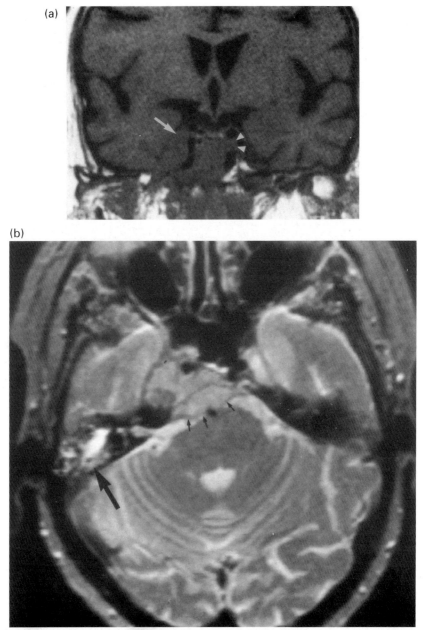

Fig. 5.9 'Aggressive' adenoma. Coronal T1-weighted MRI (**a**) and transverse T2-weighted MRI (**b**) scans. A mass arising within the sella is invading the cavernous sinuses (arrowheads, **a**), more so on the right side, and is destroying the right petrous temporal apex (arrowed). Posterior extension of the tumour is compressing the right side of the brain stem (small arrows, **b**) and displacing the basilar artery. Retained secretions are present in the mastoid air cells. This more aggressive type of adenoma is uncommon and may simulate meningioma or secondary deposit.

(a)

(b)

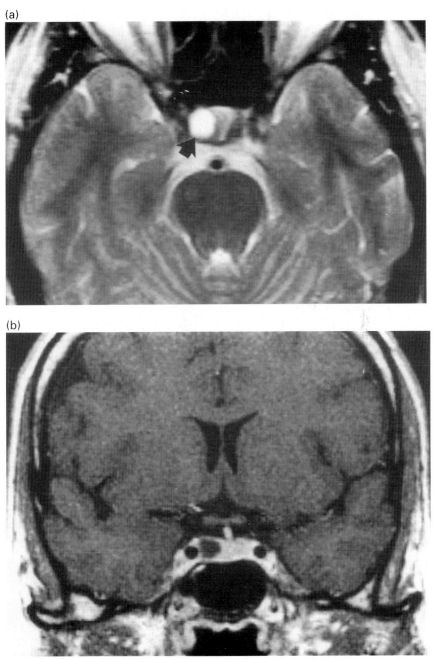

Fig. 5.10 Cystic microadenoma. Transverse T2-weighted MRI (**a**) and coronal T1-weighted image with enhancement (**b**). A 6 mm macroadenoma is situated within the right lobe of the gland (arrowed), causing very minor deviation of the pituitary stalk to the left side. The tumour is more homogeneous and of very low intensity on T1-weighted and high signal on T2-weighted due to cystic change within the tumour.

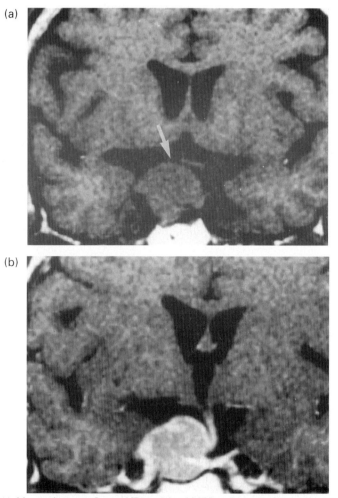

Fig. 5.11 Macroadenoma. Coronal T1-weighted MRI at the level of the optic chiasm (**a**) and after contrast through the pituitary stalk (**b**). A large mass is filling the enlarged pituitary fossa and no normal residual gland is visible. The stalk is displaced towards the left side and the floor of the sella is depressed, more on the right. The tumour shows supresellar extension which is impinging on the right side of the optic chiasma (arrowed).

Following infarction of a macroadenoma, the infarcted portion of the tumour is of lower signal intensity and does not enhance with gadolinium on T1-weighted images when compared with the viable tumour. On T2-weighted images, the infarcted tissue is relatively hyperintense compared with surrounding tissue. Following haemorrhage (Fig. 5.13), the signal characteristics follow the same temporal sequence as with intracerebral haemorrhage and initially blood is iso-intense on T1-weighted images and hypointense on T2-weighted images relative to the pituitary substance and

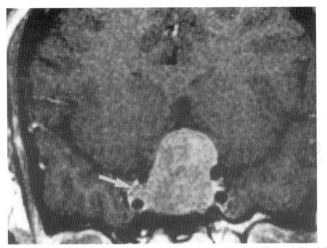

Fig. 5.12 Macroadenoma with cavernous sinus invasion. Coronal T1-weighted MRI after contrast. This large macroadenoma with an extensive suprasellar component shows invasion into the cavernous sinus on the right where tumour is seen interposed between the superior and inferior parts of the carotid syphon (arrowed).

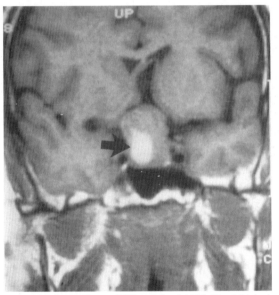

Fig. 5.13 Pituitary haemorrhage. Coronal T1-weighted MRI. Focal high signal (arrowed) is present within an enlarged gland which shows suprasellar expansion.

adenoma. When treated conservatively, the mass shows gradual involution (Fig. 5.14).[22]

Postoperatively interpretation of MR images of the pituitary is complicated by the effects of surgery and the presence of implanted materials

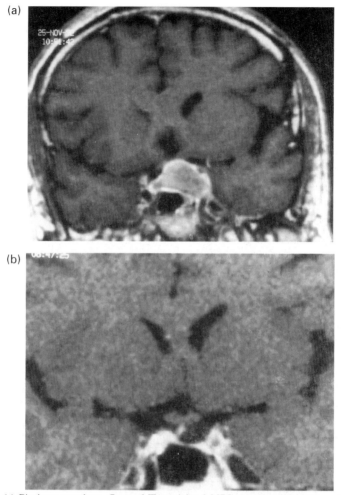

Fig. 5.14 Pituitary apoplexy. Coronal T1-weighted MRI at presentation (**a**) and 6 months later (**b**) in a 48-year-old man presenting with severe pain in the eye. A hyperintense, well-defined mass due to haemorrhage into a pituitary tumour is filling the fossa and extending to touch the chiasma. The cavernous segment of the carotid artery is bowed laterally by the mass but otherwise shows normal anatomy. Six months later the gland has atrophied and very little residual tissue is seen within the fossa. The stalk is displaced towards the right side of the fossa.

(Fig. 5.15).[23] The gland itself may appear normal or it may remain distorted or displaced; re-expansion of the gland occurs in some cases following excision of tumour. It is not possible to differentiate small residual tumours from scar tissue and implant tissues in some cases. Larger recurrentnes and residual tumour are seen due to their mass. The signal characteristics and enhancement features are variable and depend on the presence of haemorrhage and necrosis within the mass. Implant materials have variable appearances. Muscle and fat implants are inhomogeneous on MR. Gelatine

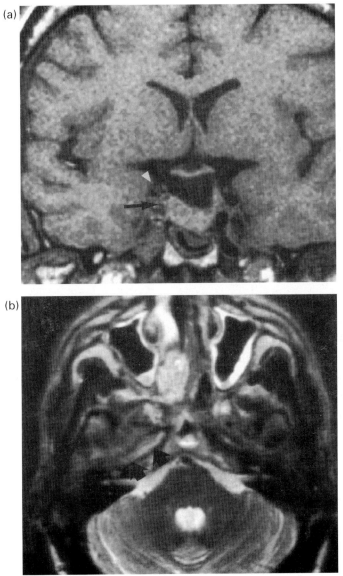

Fig. 5.15 Residual adenoma following embolization of and surgery to the right internal carotid artery for post-traumatic aneurysm. Coronal T1-weighted MRI (**a**), transverse T2-weighted MRI (**b**). A residual mass is seen in the floor of an enlarged pituitary fossa. Artifact is generated from embolization coils (arrowed). Absence of flow void (arrowhead, **a**) and high signal on T2-weighted MRI (arrowed, **b**) is seen in the right carotid artery due to thrombosis of the vessel (see also Fig. 6.15a, b).

foam implants appear as endosellar masses and may either be of homogeneous signal, isointense to grey matter or heterogeneous high signal. A
rim of peripheral enhancement (probably due to surrounding inflammatory
tissue) is commonly seen. Both the bulk of the implant and the enhancing
rim may decrease with time.

Rathke cleft cysts

Embryologically the anterior pituitary develops from a pharyngeal diverticulum which extends cranially from the mouth cavity to fuse with a diverticulum extending from the floor of the brain which forms the posterior
pituitary. Rathke cleft cysts form from remnants of the pharyngeal pouch
and may occur anywhere along its course. The majority are entirely intrasellar, some have a suprasellar component and others are entirely suprasellar;
rarely they may present as a pharyngeal mass. They have a variety of appearances depending on the cyst contents.[24] The simplest are thin walled and
contain serous fluid, hence have the signal characteristics of CSF
(Fig. 5.16). Mucoid-containing cysts are hyperintense on T1-weighted
image and iso- or hyperintense on T2-weighted scans.[24-26] Cysts containing
desquamated cellular debris have heterogeneous appearances and these
latter two types of cysts may be confused with cystic craniopharyngiomas,
although the absence of enhancement favours a Rathke's cyst. The presence
of methaemoglobin within the cyst following haemorrhage causes hyperintensity on both T1 and T2-weighted images.[27]

Rarely cysts have a thin wall of calcification but this is not visible on MR
and well shown on CT scans. Rathke's cysts may be associated with a
persistent bony canal within the sphenoid; however, this is better shown on
CT than by MR.

Craniopharyngiomas

Craniopharyngiomas may present at any age, but they are by far the commonest type of tumour affecting the pituitary/hypothalamic region in childhood and account for 8–13% of all intracranial tumours under 14 years of
age. They usually originate in the suprasellar region and form non-invasive
slowly expanding masses impinging upon the sella and enlarging it. Postero-
superior extension displaces the hypothalamus and midbrain. Inferior
extension behind the clivus may even reach through the foramen magnum.
Subfrontal and medial temporal extensions also occur, sometimes extending
through the Sylvian fissure(s) to reach the cerebral convexity(ies). Less
commonly, craniopharyngiomas arise within the sella, causing expansion
simulating a pituitary adenoma; rarely they may be infrasellar or originate
within the third ventricle.

Craniopharyngiomas may be cystic or solid, but commonly contain both
elements (Fig. 5.17). Less commonly they may be entirely solid or be

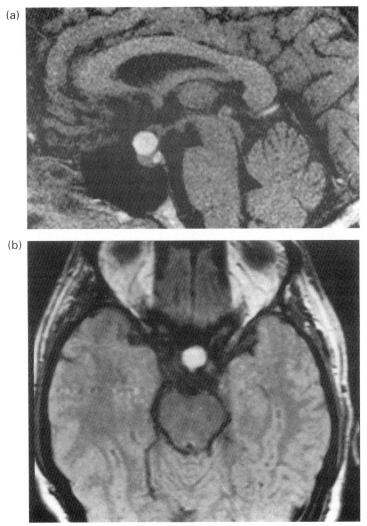

Fig. 5.16 Rathke's cleft cyst. Sagittal (**a**) and transverse PD-weighted (**b**) images. A 10 mm well-defined hyperintense mass on T1 and PD weighting is lying anterior to the pituitary stalk, displacing the gland inferiorly and touching the chiasma superiorly. Normal posterior and anterior pituitary tissue is seen within the sella. The signal within the tumour is homogeneous. Although hyperintensity is the most common signal pattern in these tumours they may also be iso- or hypointense compared with brain substance on T1 or T2 weighting.

represented by an entirely calcified mass. Both solid and cystic components of the tumour are hyperintense on T2-weighted images and reliable separation of these elements is not possible using this sequence. The appearances are more variable in T1-weighted images and tumours may be hyper-, iso- or hypointense compared to grey matter. Hyperintensity on T1-weighted images is related to the presence of high protein, calcification and/or

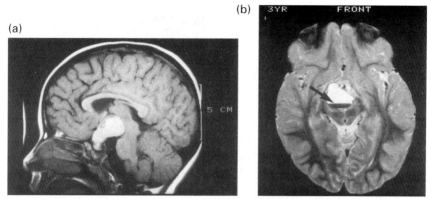

Fig. 5.17 Craniopharyngioma. Sagittal T1-weighted MRI (**a**), transverse T2-weighted MRI (**b**). A predominantly suprasellar well-defined smooth-walled tumour is displacing the brain stem posteriorly, lifting the floor of the third ventricle and extending into the pituitary fossa. The tumour is almost entirely cystic and has characteristic high signal on T1, probably due to protein within the fluid. A fluid level on the transverse scan (arrowed, **b**) confirms the cyst. The low signal in the lower fluid is probably due to haemosiderin.

methaemoglobin and not the concentration of cholesterol triglycerides.[28] Fluid levels may be seen within the cysts in some cases (Fig. 5.17). As with CT, enhancement may be helpful in defining the structure of the tumours, as solid portions of the tumour generally enhance with contrast. The cyst wall, but not the contents, may enhance.

Calcification (which may be rim or nodular) is present in over 90% of childhood craniopharyngiomas and it contributes to the heterogeneous appearance of the tumour (Fig. 5.18). Occasionally dense calcification is seen as regions of signal void. Potentially small, densely calcified tumours may be missed on MR when they would be comparatively easy to identify on CT.[29] In low concentrations, it may return non-specific T1 high signal but it may not be identified on MRI when clearly visible on CT. Since calcification may be significant in suggesting a specific diagnosis or important in identifying small tumours, either initially or following surgery, CT may be indicated if the findings on MRI are negative or equivocal.

Uncommonly craniopharyngiomas behave as invasive tumours infiltrating brain substance and causing reactive oedema. The latter may spread along the direction of fibre tracts and extend in a manner simulating an optic glioma.

Large craniopharyngiomas may obstruct the CSF pathways causing hydrocephalus or present acutely due to sudden expansion of cystic components, sometimes due to haemorrhagic changes.

Germ cell tumours

These constitute about 1% of intracranial tumours. They are mainly situated in the pineal region, but about 20% occur in the suprasellar/pituitary region, where they may be primary or due to transventricular spread from the pineal.

(a) (b)

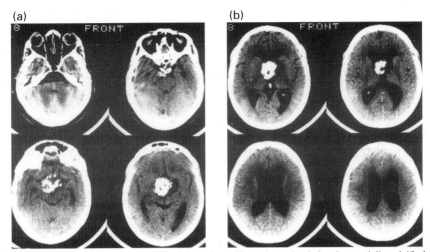

Fig. 5.18 Craniopharyngioma. CT axial sections. There is a mixed-density partially calcified mass with a cystic component in the medial part of the left middle fossa. The mass involves the pontine, chiasmatic and interventricular cisterns and extends superiorly through the third ventricle to encroach on the frontal horns and occlude the foramen of Monro, causing hydrocephalus with periventricular lucency.

(a) (b)

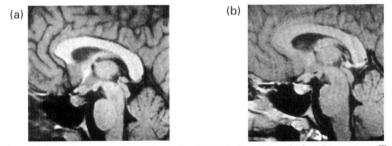

Fig. 5.19 Germinoma. Sagittal T1-weighted MRI before (**a**) and after (**b**) contrast. Tumour infiltration is causing thickening of the tuber cinereum and pituitary stalk and absence of high signal in the posterior pituitary in this child suffering from diabetes insipidus.

Germ cell tumours are subdivided into germinomatous (GGCT 65%), which rarely produce tumour markers, and non-germinomatous germ cell tumours (NGGCT), in which α-fetoprotein and/or chorionic gonadatrophin in the CSF are commonly present, and may give some indication of the histological composition of this more malignant subgroup. The tumours occur in childhood and have a marked male preponderance. GGCT are well-defined homogeneous masses of T1 low, T2 high signal on MRI and of greater than brain density on CT without calcification in the tumour matrix. They show intense uniform enhancement (Fig. 5.19). They are generally well demarcated from the adjacent structures in the early stages, but they tend to infiltrate or extend along the walls of the third ventricle in

(a)   (b)

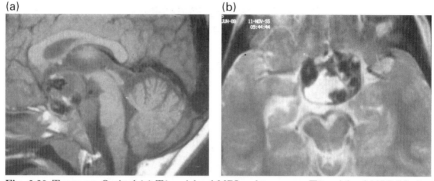

Fig. 5.20 Teratoma. Sagittal (**a**) T1-weighted MRI and transverse T2-weighted MRI (**b**). A well-circumscribed mixed-intensity mass containing several teeth (T1 and T2 low signal) and fat (T1 high signal). The mass occupies the chiasmatic and pontine cisterns, with the optic chiasm lying anteriorly and the pituitary compressed beneath it.

more advanced cases. Haemorrhage into the tumour is not uncommon and metastatic spread within the ventricles and subarachnoid space is frequent. The tumour responds rapidly to radiotherapy and may be cured.

NGGCT may show calcification within the tumour matrix and tend to undergo cystic, haemorrhagic and necrotic changes resulting in a hetero-geneous appearance with irregular enhancement. Well-differentiated teratomas, which are a subgroup of NGGCT, also form heterogeneous masses. There are enhancing soft tissue components similar to brain in CT density and MR signal with additional regions containing fat, calcification, ossification or occasionally tooth formation (Fig. 5.20). Haemorrhage is common in these tumours and contributes to the heterogeneous appearance. As well as producing suprasellar mass effects and endocrine symptoms secondary to specific hormone secretions, the tumour may rupture with leakage of fat globules, which may remain free within the CSF spaces, but tend to become fixed and may cause a chemical reaction associated with adhesion formation and hydrocephalus. The NGGCT respond incom-pletely and temporarily to radiation, but prognosis has been markedly improved by chemotherapy.

Epidermoids and dermoids

These benign embryonic inclusions may present as suprasellar masses. Epi-dermoids most frequently form masses of approximately CSF density on CT and may simulate arachnoid cysts, although they are generally more irregular in shape (Fig. 5.21) On T1-weighted sequences, the signal returned is generally low, tending to approximate to that of CSF. The signal may be similar to CSF on T2-weighted sequences also, although it is usually a little higher, and the differential intensity from CSF on proton density sequences is generally sufficient to allow the margins of the tumour to be defined

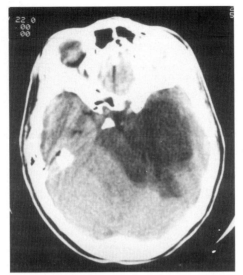

Fig. 5.21 Epidermoid. Cranial CT. There is a large low-density loublated mass in the left middle fossa, chiasmatic, interpeduncular, pontine and ambiens cisterns, displacing the midbrain and temporal lobe. The density is similar to CSF and apart from the prominent lobulation the mass could have been an arachnoid cyst.

(Fig. 5.22). Occasionally, there is calcification in the tumour capsule, which may also show a thin rim of enhancement. Suprasellar epidermoids may show a frond-like infiltration into the middle fossa or temporal horn, causing a virtually pathognomonic appearance; such extension may be associated with complex partial seizures.

Intracranial dermoids are rare, but the suprasellar region is second in incidence as their site of origin only to the pineal. Like epidermoids, they may present with chiasmal compression or endocrine disturbances including delayed growth or precocious puberty. On both CT and MRI they may be recognized as well-demarcated masses containing fat in association with other soft tissues in which enhancement may be patchy or absent (Fig. 4.23) They tend to be smaller than teratomas and rapid growth and surrounding oedema distinguish the latter. Lipomas also occur in this region as well-defined small masses composed of fat alone without the other tissues associated with the inclusion tumour group. Suprasellar lipomas are discovered incidentally and are asymptomatic lesions which require no further investigation.

Chiasmatic and hypothalamic gliomas

Optic gliomas usually present with disturbances of vision and hypothalamic tumours with precocious puberty in males or with symptoms of hypothalamic disturbance, diabetes insipidus or pituitary insufficiency.

(a)

(b)

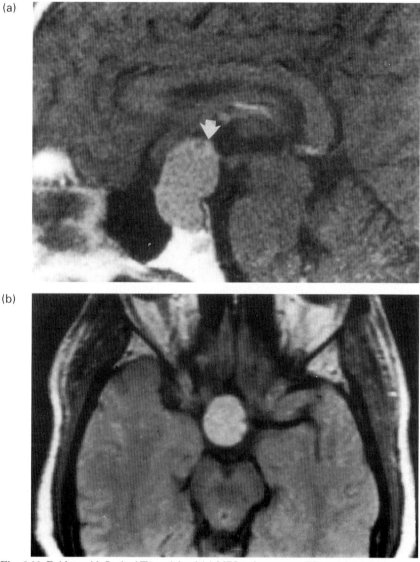

Fig. 5.22 Epidermoid. Sagittal T1-weighted (**a**) MRI and transverse PD-weighted (**b**) images. The tumour is of intermediate intensity on T1 and characteristically hyperintense on PD-weighted images. The sella is enlarged and the mass is elevating the floor of the third ventricle (arrowed). No normal pituitary stalk or gland is visible.

Optic gliomas are usually low-grade astrocytomas and they account for about 5% of intracranial tumours presenting before the age of 10 years. The tumour may be more malignant, particularly if it presents at a relatively older age. It may involve the chiasm alone, but it tends to extend along and expand the optic tract(s) and/or optic nerve(s), tending to maintain the

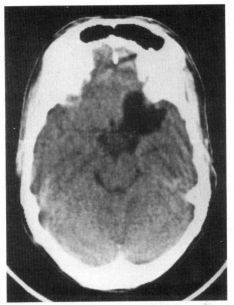

Fig. 5.23 Dermoid. Transverse CT. There is a clearly defined mass in the left chiasmatic, sylvian and subfrontal regions. It is of mainly lower density than CSF but higher density than the air in the frontal sinus, indicating that it contains fat which could be within a lipoma or a dermoid. The situation would be most unusual for the former and at operation a dermoid was resected.

anatomical features of the optic apparatus (Figs 5.24 and 5.25). Invasion of adjacent structures may occur and the origin of the tumour may then be in doubt.

Gliomas of the hypothalamus also tend to be of low grade, and like the optic glioma have an MR T1 signal usually similar to that of normal white matter. On T2 the signal is generally higher than brain substance. Enhancement is usual (Fig. 5.26), although it may be only minor or moderate in degree. Cystic changes may be present.

Mestastases in the suprasellar region

These occur from pineal germ cell tumours, from medulloblastomas and retinoblastomas. They may present with endocrine upset, but the primary tumour is usually evident at the time of diagnosis with gadolinium-enhanced sagittal MRI. Metastases from systemic tumours also occur to the surrounding bony structures (Fig. 5.27) or to the pituitary stalk and the pituitary gland itself (Fig. 5.28). The former present with diabetes insipidus and the latter simulate a non-endocrine tumour of the pituitary gland itself. The most usual primary is carcinoma of the breast or bronchus and the chest X-

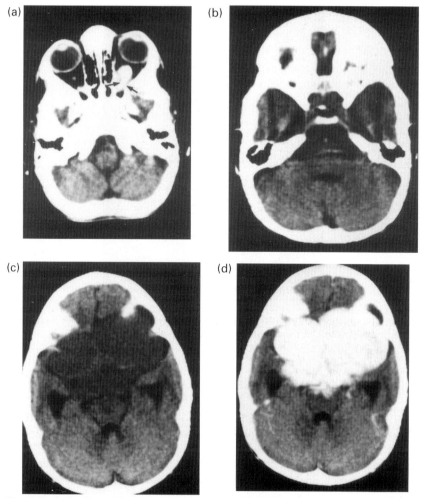

Fig. 5.24 Optic glioma. Transverse CT scans before (a–c) and after (d) contrast enhancement. There is a large low-density (c) enhancing (d) mass in the optic chiasm eroding the tuberculum sellae and chiasmatic sulcus and enlarging the left optic nerve (arrowed, **a**).

ray is likely to be abnormal at the time of presentation of the intracranial tumour.

Parasellar meningioma

These lesions usually present with visual or oculomotor disturbances, but hypopituitarism is not uncommon. Meningiomas extending into the sella may originate from the planum sphenoidale, the sphenoidal wing or anterior clinoid process, tuberculum sellae, dorsum sellae, the diaphragm itself or the dura lining the cavernous sinuses. There is usually a distinct plane of

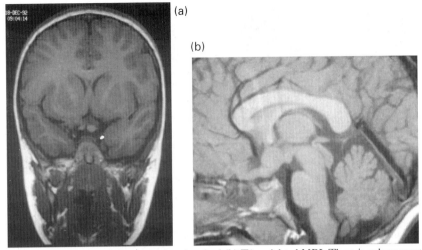

Fig. 5.25 Optic glioma. Coronal (**a**) and sagittal (**b**) T1-weighted MRI. There is enlargement of the left optic nerve (**a**) and left side of the optic chiasm (**b**) where tumour is crossing the midline.

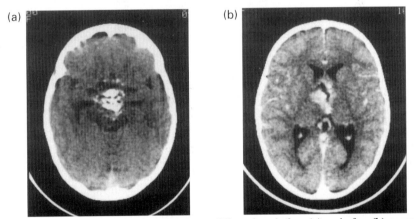

Fig. 5.26 Hypothalamic glioma. Transverse CT sections before (**a**) and after (**b**) contrast enhancement. There is a partly calcified enhancing mass in the hypothalamus. It obliterates the chiasmatic cistern and fills the region of the third ventricle (see also Fig. 9.10).

demarcation, usually a dural partition between the meningioma and the pituitary substance. Meningiomas tend to be isointense with grey matter on T1-weighted sequences and iso- or hyperintense on moderately T2-weighted and hyperintense on heavily T2-weighted sequences: they tend to enhance markedly (Fig. 5.29). The tumours usually have a broad dural base, the adjacent bone may show hyperostosis and psammomatous calcification within the meningioma is frequent. Encasement of the arteries causing

(a)   (b)

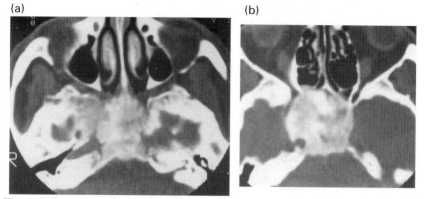

Fig. 5.27 Parasellar bone metastasis from carcinoma of prostate. Axial (**a, b**) CT. Irregular mixed low and mainly high density in the sphenoid bone is encroaching on the sella.

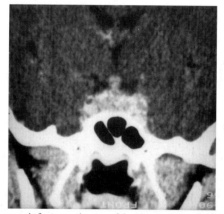

Fig. 5.28 Pituitary metastasis from carcinoma of the breast. Coronal CT section after enhancement. The pituitary gland is enlarged and there is thickening of the pituitary stalk by metastasis to the gland.

narrowing of the lumen is typical of meningioma but occurs with a relatively lesser frequency in pituitary adenomas.

Parasellar schwannomas

These lesions arise from the nerves passing through the cavernous sinus or their pre- or post-cavernous segments. They rarely simulate a pituitary lesion and do not cause endocrine effects. Occasionally they cause nodular masses, which can impinge upon pituitary substance, but are demarcated from it by the dura lining the pituitary fossa. They are T1 low, T2 high signal-enhancing lesions, which can usually be specifically identified by their relationship to the course of the involved cranial nerve.

(a)

(b)

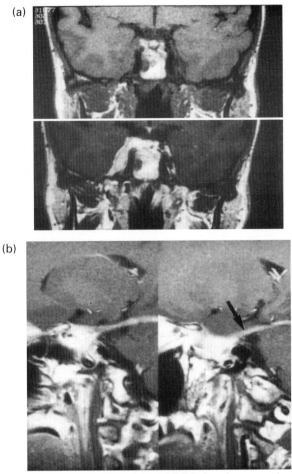

Fig. 5.29 Meningioma. Coronal T1-weighted MRI before (**a**, upper picture) and after (**a**, lower picture) enhancement and sagittal T1-weighted image after contrast (**b**). There is enlargement and abnormal enhancement of the right cavernous sinus, thickening of the medial border of the right side of the middle fossa and tentorial margin (arrowed). There is abnormal enhancement of these regions (see also Fig. 10.1).

Chordomas and chondromas

Tumours arising from the skull base include chordoma and chondroma, which are generally recognized as a group from the bone destruction, sometimes combined with expansion, which is constant. They may remain entirely extradural, causing mass effect, displacing the dura, and tending to elevate or compress the structures contained within the dura, which may include the pituitary gland. Erosion through the dura is not uncommon, particularly with larger chordomas. It is evident on imaging if the edge of the tumour encroaching into the CSF or on the intradural structures is irregular. It is much more frequent with neoplastic recurrence following surgery which has breached the dura.

Chordomas are tumours derived from the remnants of the primitive notochord and in the cranium are found almost exclusively in the clivus. Rarely they may be found in the pituitary fossa or in the petrous bone. When situated in the sella or parasellar regions the tumours present with symptoms due to their mass effect, to pituitary insufficiency or to invasion of the cavernous sinuses. Chordomas typically cause bone destruction. The matrix of a chondroma usually contains calcification or ossification and they are frequently gelatinous or semi-liquid on macroscopic examination. Chordomas vary in consistency between a soft, almost mucoid and a fibrous matrix. On MR, chordomas appear as iso- or hypointense masses on T1- and of moderate to high signal on T2-weighted sequences (see Fig. 10.3, Parasellar chapter).[30] The mucoid substance of the tumour is of higher intensity on T2-weighted images, with the fibrous septa traversing the tumours seen as low signal strands. Enhancement is usual, though it may be slight, and vascularity varies markedly.

Although MR is better for showing the extent of the tumours and their relationship to adjacent structures, the bony destruction and tumour calcification are seen more clearly on CT scans.

Vascular Lesions

Aneurysms

Aneurysms arising within or extending into the subarachnoid space may present with subarachnoid haemorrhage, or as compressive lesions affecting adjacent cranial nerves or other structures including the pituitary infundibulum or hypothalamus. Aneurysms arising within a cavernous sinus generally present as mass lesions compressing the cranial nerves and eroding the adjacent parts of the sphenoid bone. Rupture results in 'spontaneous' caroticocavernous fistulas which, like post-traumatic direct fistulas, present with bruit, chemosis and oculomotor paresis, which can be of neurogenic or myogenic origin. The anatomy of patent vessels is well shown on MRI due to the vessels being outlined by flow void or flow-related enhancement. The vascular anatomy can be further documented using MR angiography. The signal returned from thrombus within vessels varies with the age of the clot, but high signal return from methaemoglobin may partly fill an aneurysmal lumen (Fig. 5.30), sometimes with a layered effect due to recurrent bleeding into the thrombus within the wall of the aneurysm. Dilatation of the cavernous sinus and superior ophthalmic vein is usually associated with congestion, causing enlargement of the extrinsic muscles of the orbit.

Dural arteriovenous malformations and fistulas cause similar pathognomonic but much less marked signs of arteriovenous shunting with congestion of orbital structures. Dural fistulas in particular may be com-

(a) (b)

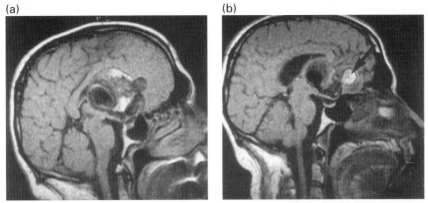

Fig. 5.30 Giant anterior communicating aneurysm. Sagittal T1-weighted MRI. There is a large lobulated mass in the subfrontal regions displacing the optic chiasm inferiorly, the third ventricle posteriorly and the corpus callosum posterosuperiorly. The mass returns mixed signal, one loculus of the periphery (arrowed) being high due to clot containing methaemoglobin and other parts of the tumour being low due to continuing arterial flow and turbulence.

plicated by venous sinus thrombosis, causing an absence of the flow void within the affected sinus and its replacement by high signal due to slow flow-related enhancement or to methaemoglobin within recent thrombus.

Pituitary apoplexy

Due to infarction of the gland with or without haemorrhage into the gland substance apoplexy usually occurs in association with macroadenomas, sometimes following bromocriptine therapy. Necrotic and haemorrhagic foci within adenomas are not infrequent, but classic pituitary apoplexy presents with sudden headache, oculomotor paresis or visual impairment due to chiasmatic compression. The headache may suggest subarachnoid haemorrhage, sometimes due to subarachnoid extension of the bleeding. The condition is simply diagnosed from the presence of high signal methaemoglobin on T1- and T2-weighted sequences within or replacing the macroadenoma (Figure 5.14). CT high density may also be present, but haemorrhage is recognized in only about 25% of the lesions in which it is shown by MRI.

Metabolic

Diabetes insipidus

Diabetes insipidus (DI) may be caused either by primary failure of production of antidiuretic hormone by the cells of the paraventricular nuclei, or by destruction of the hypothalamus or of the axons from it linking through the infundibulum to the posterior pituitary secondary to a variety of disorders including tumours, trauma or inflammatory conditions, and the radiological appearances reflect this. In all cases of central DI and some of nephrogenic DI, the high signal normally present in the posterior portion of the gland on T1-weighted images is absent. This is a useful distinguishing feature from primary polydipsia in which the high signal is maintained. This may be the only finding in primary DI.[31] As this finding may occur in under 10% of normal individuals, too much weight must not be put on this observation in the absence of biochemical disturbance. Following trauma, the pituitary stalk may appear transected or thinned with accumulation of high signal on the T1-weighted image proximal to the transected stalk or within the hypothalamus. This is thought to represent accumulation of neurosecretory vesicles proximal to the damaged portion of the stalk.

In DI due to other causes, the MR findings are primarily those of the underlying pathology, e.g. germinoma (see above).

Pre- and post-gadolinium T1-weighted sections in both coronal and sagittal planes are necessary for the diagnosis of lesions causing central DI. Very small neoplastic or inflammatory lesions may be responsible, and if the diagnosis is not apparent the CSF should be examined for α-fetoprotein and human gonadotrophin. When negative, the imaging should be repeated at intervals of less than 1 year when the DI persists.

Haemochromatosis

Haemochromatosis is associated with heavy deposition of haemosiderin in many tissues, including the pituitary gland. The condition is associated with pituitary insufficiency. The ferric iron produces susceptibility effects causing marked loss of signal from the pituitary gland on T2-weighted sequences. This is a pathognomonic sign of the condition, although it is rarely of diagnostic value because the condition is clinically evident.

Tumour-like conditions of the sellar and parasellar regions

Arachnoid cysts

Symptomatic arachnoid cysts usually present in infancy with hydrocephalus or in early life as compressive mass lesions with visual loss, hypopituitarism or with seizures. More frequently, they are seen as incidental findings on imaging. An intra- or parasellar location is seen in about 15% of all arachnoid cysts, which are most commonly located in the anterior third of the middle cranial fossa.[32]

Suprasellar arachnoid cysts are believed to occur developmentally as a consequence of an imperforate membrane of Liliequist with the resulting formation of a CSF-filled diverticulum.[33]

The cyst wall is usually composed of connective tissue with arachnoid cells and the cyst contents may be proteinaceous and contain pituitary hormones.[35]

On MRI, the cysts are typically well defined with contents that display signal intensities identical to that of CSF on T1, T2 and proton density-weighted images.[32,35] The adjacent brain may be displaced if the cyst is large but will display normal signal intensities. There may also be some remodelling of the skull base with larger cysts. There will be no calcification or soft tissue masses associated with the cyst and no enhancement with gadolinium. These features help to distinguish them from the main radio-logical differential diagnoses, which include epidermoids, craniopharyn-giomas and parasitic cysts.

Hypothalamic hamartomas

Clinically symptomatic lesions in these suprasellar tumours are associated with precocious puberty and seizures, but vision is usually unimpaired and focal neurological signs absent. They are usually composed of tissues of neural origin but may also contain mesenchymal elements and are typically seen in the midline as sessile or pedunculated masses. The posterior hypo-thalamus is usually affected, particularly the pituitary stalk, tuber cinereum and mamillary bodies.

The anatomical location of these lesions is demonstrated well on sagittal or coronal MRI. The tumours are isointense with grey matter on T1-weighted images but may be iso- or hyperintense compared to grey matter on T2-weighted images (Fig. 5.31). Important distinguishing features include the lack of enhancement and no evidence of growth or local invasion on follow-up. Calcification, fat, cyst formation and contrast enhancement have all been reported but are unusual findings.[36,37]

Langerhans cell histiocytosis

This embraces a spectrum of granulomatous diseases in which Langerhans cells migrate to sites outside the epidermis and cause soft tissue damage, probably mediated by excess production of cytokines and prostaglandins.[38] It typically affects children or young adults. Involvement of the sellar and parasellar regions has been described in all of the three major clinical groups of eosinophilic granuloma, Hans–Schüller–Christian disease and Letterer–Siwe disease. Histologically, the granulomas demonstrate a proliferation of histiocytes with vesicular or lobulated basophilic nucleoli and bear inclusions called X-bodies. There is often an infiltration of lymphocytes, plasma cells and eosinophils, and tissue necrosis.

The classical clinical triad in Hans–Schüller–Christian disease of exophthalmos, DI and lytic bone defects is seen in only about 25% of cases. Granulomas are seen to involve the hypothalamus, pituitary stalk and less often the pituitary gland by infiltration and thickening in about 50% of

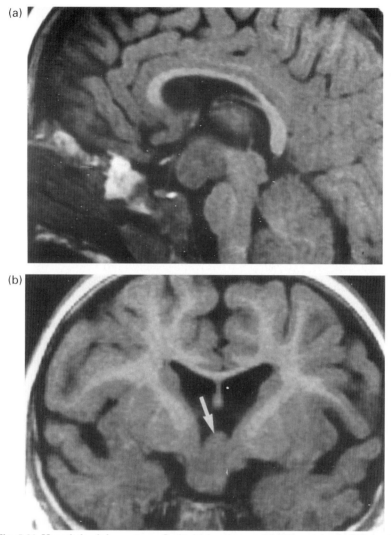

Fig. 5.31 Hypothalamic hamartoma. Sagittal (**a**) and coronal (**b**) T1-weighted MRI. A midline tumour is arising from the hypothalamus lying posterior to the pituitary stalk and lifting the floor of the third ventricle (arrowed). These tumours may be hypointense (as in this case) or isointense with grey matter.

cases. The pathogenesis of pituitary dysfunction in the other 50% is poorly understood but is presumed to be a toxic effect of substances from Langerhans cells, which may also account for white matter lesions. Symmetrical T2 high, T1 low signal regions in the white matter, most commonly involving the cerebellum, are occasional accompanying lesions. On MRI the granulomas are hyperintense on T2-weighted imaging and enhance with gadolinium. In cases with diabetes insipidus, the normal high signal of the

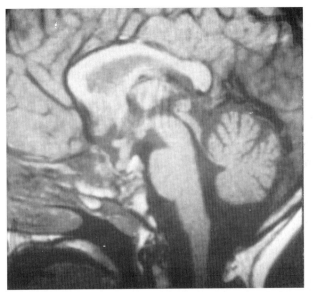

Fig. 5.32 Histiocytosis. Sagittal T1-weighted MRI after contrast. The pituitary stalk is abnormally thickened and shows enhancement. The normal high signal within the posterior pituitary was absent in this child presenting with diabetes insipidus. Further deposits are present within the sella.

posterior pituitary on T1-weighted images is absent (Fig. 5.32). Lytic destruction of the sphenoid bone with eosinophilic granuloma and Letterer–Siwe disease may also occur. Diagnosis is usually by biopsy of an accessible bone lesion. Lesions may be treated with local curettage or radiotherapy and systemic steroids with or without adjuvant chemotherapy.

Infective and inflammatory conditions of the sellar and parasellar regions

Sellar and parasellar infections

Bacterial infections are rare and may occur by local spread from the paranasal sinuses or meninges or may have spread haematogenously from more distant foci. Infections occurring as a complication of surgery are very rare.

Pituitary abscesses typically present with headache, visual loss and pituitary dysfunction. With the exception of pyrexia, systemic manifestations are uncommon. There is an association with coexisting disease of the sellar or parasellar regions such as pituitary adenomas, craniopharyngiomas or Rathke's cleft cysts.[39] The commonest organisms are Gram-positive cocci.

Unenhanced MRI will reveal lesions that are indistinguishable from pituitary adenomas. Ring enhancement with a fluid centre is seen following intravenous gadolinium. There may be a fluid level in the sphenoid sinus.[40]

Tuberculous involvement of the sellar and parasellar regions is uncommon. It typically occurs by extension of the infection from the basal meninges. A granulomatous nodular enhancement pattern is seen on imaging. On the development of tuberculomas, fairly characteristic patterns of MR signals may be seen. Early immature tuberculomas are small with central areas of necrosis and a fibrous peripheral rim of granulation tissue. On T2-weighted imaging there is central high signal with an iso- or hypointense rim surrounded by hyperintense oedema. On T1-weighted imaging, there is a hypointense core with a rim that is isointense with grey matter. Larger, more mature tuberculomas excite less reactive oedema as they form a dense peripheral wall of granulation and compressed glial tissue. They have a more solid appearance with 'growth rings' of deposited granulation tissue. This fibrous peripheral rim appears hypointense on T2 imaging and isointense on T1 imaging.[41]

Similarly, congenital or acquired syphilis of the pituitary is now rare and is more often diagnosed at post-mortem or by the concurrence of pituitary dysfunction and serological evidence of syphilis.[42]

Parasitic infestations such as cysticercosis have been reported to involve the parasellar regions. The diagnosis is usually evident from the involvement by disease elsewhere and with the typical MR appearance of the cysticercus: that of a vesicle with a high-intensity nodule inside the sphere which corresponds to the scolex.[43]

Infection of the cavernous sinus leading to thrombosis may occur secondary to venous septic emboli draining from periorbital or paranasal disease.

Sarcoid

Neurological involvement in sarcoid occurs in about 5% of cases, with cranial nerve palsies being the commonest presentation. Involvement of the sellar and parasellar regions leads to DI and hypopituitarism which may have an indolent and progressive course.

The diagnosis is usually made on the systemic manifestations of this chronic, multisystem disorder, although a rare case of juxtasellar disease in the absence of systemic disease has been reported.[44] The histological hallmark is that of the non-caseating granuloma on biopsy of an accessible lesion or lymph node.

Radiologically, there are usually multiple enhancing nodules or masses in the meninges and along the cranial nerves. Heterogenous nodular infiltrations into the brain parenchyma may occur along the Virchow–Robin spaces with surrounding reactive oedema. Lesions are usually hypointense on T1-weighted imaging but may display a variety of signal intensities on T2-weighted imaging, with hyperintensity most commonly seen.[45] In pituitary and hypothalamic disease causing DI, the normal high signal of the posterior pituitary on T1-weighted imaging will be absent (Fig. 5.33).

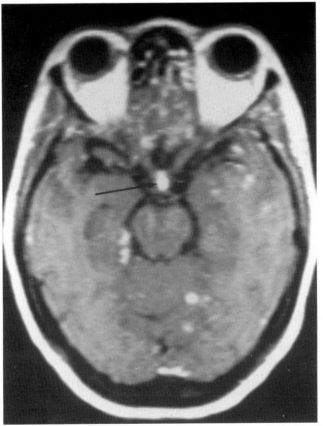

Fig. 5.33 Sarcoid. CT scan after contrast. An enhancing granuloma is sited in the pituitary stalk (arrowed). Further granulomas are seen elsewhere in the brain parenchyma and meninges.

Tolosa–Hunt syndrome

This is a syndrome of steroid-responsive painful ophthalmoplegia associated with an inflammatory lesion of the cavernous sinus. Pathologically, there is a similarity to orbital pseudotumours and histologically it is seen to contain fibroblasts, plasma cells and lymphocytes. Involvement of other nerves in the cavernous sinus is common and although the disease is self-limiting, irreversible damage may occur.[46]

Abnormal soft tissue is seen to infiltrate an enlarged cavernous sinus and often extends to reach the orbital apex. The intracavernous carotid artery may be irregularly constricted. Thrombosis of the cavernous sinus and superior ophthalmic vein is a reported complication.[47] The soft tissue is isointense with muscle on T1-weighted imaging and isointense with fat on T2-weighted imaging. A prompt and dramatic response to steroid therapy is a major diagnostic feature.

(a)   (b)

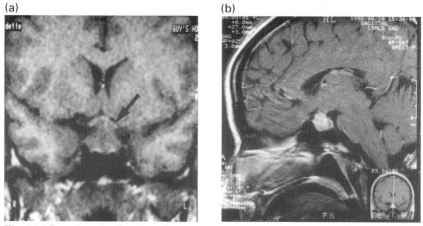

Fig. 5.34 Lymphocytic adenohypophysitis. Coronal T1-weighted image before (**a**) and sagittal T1-weighted image after contrast (**b**). There is diffuse enlargement of the pituitary gland which shows intense enhancement. There is suprasellar extension of the gland which is lifting the optic chiasm (arrowed).

Lymphocytic adenohypophysitis

This inflammatory condition of the anterior pituitary occurs almost exclusively in women in late pregnancy or early in the post-partum period. The clinical presentation is that of headache and visual loss, with a failure to resume menses or a failure to lactate, and hypopituitarism.

Typically there is a homogeneous inflammatory mass infiltrating and enlarging the anterior pituitary that is histologically composed of lymphocytes, plasma cells and fibrosis surrounding islands of hyperplastic lactotrophs. The diffuse pituitary gland enlargement usually extends into the suprasellar region, with no focal changes seen in the internal signal characteristics of the gland (Fig. 5.34). There is believed to be an autoimmune aetiology and the condition is associated with Hashimoto's thyroiditis. Antiprolactin antibodies have been identified in some cases.[48,49] The condition is steroid responsive but may regress spontaneously after delivery.

REFERENCES

1. National Radiological Protection Board. Patients dose reduction in diagnostic radiology. Doc NRPB 1990; 1: 31–32.
2. Haughton VM, Proat R. Pituitary fossa: chemical shift effect in MR imaging. Radiology 1986; 158: 461–462.
3. Fujisawa I, Nishimura K, Asato R et al. Posterior lobe of the pituitary and diabetes insipidus: MR findings. J Comput Assist Tomogr 1987; 11: 221–225.
4. Fujisawa I, Asato R, Kawata M et al. Hyperintense signal of the posterior pituitary on T1-weighted MRI: an experimental study. J Comput Assist Tomogr 1989; 13: 371–377.
5. Kim BJ, Kido DK, Simon JH et al. Chemical shift MR imaging of posterior lobe of pituitary gland (abstract). AJNR 1989; 10: 1281–1282.

6. Mark LP, Haughton VM, Hendrix LE et al. High-intensity signal within the posterior pituitary fossa: a study with fat-suppression MR techniques. AJR 1991; 157: 389–392.
7. Miki Y, Matsuo M, Nishizawa S et al. Pituitary adenomas and normal pituitary tissue: enhancement patterns on gadopentate-enhanced MR imaging. Radiology 1990; 177: 35–38.
8. Sakamoto Y, Takahashi M, Korogi Y et al. Normal and abnormal pituitary glands: gadopentate dimeglumine-enhanced MR imaging. Radiology 1991; 178: 441–445.
9. Tien RD. Sequence of enhancement of various portions of the pituitary gland on gadolinium-enhanced MR images: correlation with regional blood supply. AJR 1992; 158: 651–654.
10. Cox TD, Elster TD. Normal pituitary gland changes in shape, size and signal intensity during the first year of life of MR imaging. Radiology 1991; 179: 721–724.
11. Elster AD, Chen MYM, Williams DW, Key LL. Pituitary gland: MR imaging of physiologic hypertrophy in adolescence. Radiology 1990; 174: 681–685.
12. Doraiswamy PM, Potts JM, Figiel GS et al. MR imaging of physiological pituitary gland hypertrophy in adolescence (letter). Radiology 1991; 178: 284–285.
13. Hayakawa K, Konishi Y, Matsuda T et al. Development and aging of brain midline structures: assessment with MR imaging. Radiology 1989; 172: 171–177.
14. Suzuki M, Takashima T, Kadoya M et al. Height of normal pituitary gland on MR imaging: age and sex differentiation. J Comput Assist Tomogr 1990; 14: 36–39.
15. Elster AD, Saunders TG, Vines FS, Chen MYM. Size and shape of the pituitary gland during pregnancy and post partum: measurement with MR imaging. Radiology 1991; 181: 531–535.
16. Ferreri AJM, Garrido SA, Markarian MG, Yanz A. Relationship between the development of diaphragma sellae and the morphology of the sella turcica and its content. Surg Radiol Anat 1992; 14: 233–239.
17. Mark L, Pech P, Daniels D, Charles C, Williams A, Haughton V. The pituitary fossa: a correlative anatomic and NMR study. Radiology 1984; 153: 453–457.
18. Kelly WM, Jucharczyk W, Kuucharcyzk J et al. Posterior pituitary ectopia: an MR feature of pituitary dwarfism. AJNR 1988; 9: 453–460.
19. Diebler C, Dulac O. Cephalocoeles: clinical and neuroradiological appearance. Neuroradiology 1983; 25: 199–216.
20. Truwit CL, Barckovich AJ, Grumbach MM, Martini JJ. MR imaging of Kallman syndrome, a genetic disorder of neuronal migration affecting the olfactory and genital systems. AJNR 1993; 14: 827–838.
21. Scotti G, Yu-C-Y, Dillion WP et al. MR imaging of cavernous sinus involvement by pituitary adenomas. AJR 1988; 151: 799–806.
22. Armstrong MR, Douek M, Schellinger D, Patronas NJ. Regression of pituitary macroadenoma after pituitary apoplexy: CT and MR Studies. J Comput Assist Tomogr 1991; 15: 832–834.
23. Steiner E, Knosp E, Herold CH et al. Pituitary adenomas: findings of post-operative MR imaging. Radiology 1992; 185: 521–527.
24. Asari S, Ito T, Tsuchida S, Tsutsui T. MR appearances and cyst content of Rathke's cleft cysts. J Comput Assist Tomogr 1990; 14: 532–535.
25. Nemoto Y, Inoue Y, Fukuda T et al. MR appearance of Rathke's cleft cysts. Neuroradiology 1988; 30: 155–159.
26. Maggio WW, Cail WS, Brookeman JR, Persing JA, Jane JA. Rathke's cleft cyst: computed tomographic and magnetic resonance imaging appearances. Neurosurgery 1987; 21: 60–62.
27. Mize W, Ball WS, Towbin RB, Han BK. Atypical CT and MR appearances of a Rathke cleft cyst. Am J Neuroradiol 1989; 10: S83–S84.
28. Ahmadi J, Destian S, Aputzzo MLJ et al. Cystic fluid in craniopharyngiomas: MR imaging and quantative analysis. Radiology 1992; 182: 783–785.
29. Freeman MP, Kessler RM, Allen JH, Price AC. Craniopharyngioma: CT and MR imaging in 9 cases. J Comput Assist Tomogr 1987; 11: 810–814.
30. Sze G, Uichanco LS, Brant-Zawadski MN et al. Chordomas: MR imaging. Radiology 1988; 166: 187–191.
31. Fujisawa I, Asato R, Nishimura K et al. Anterior and posterior lobes of the pituitary gland: assessment by 1.5T MR imaging. J Comput Assist Tomogr 1987; 11: 214–220.

32. Wiener SN, Pearlstein AE, Eiber A. MR imaging of intracranial arachnoid cysts. J Comput Assist Tomogr 1987; 11: 236–241.
33. Fox JL, Al-Mefty O. Suprasellar arachnoid cysts: an extension of the membrane of Liliequist. Neurosurgery 1980; 7: 615–618.
34. Hasegawa M, Yamashima T, Yamashita J, Kuroda E. Symptomatic intrasellar arachnoid cyst: case report. Surg Neurol 1991; 35: 355–359.
35. Kjos BO, Brant-Zawadski M, Kucharczyk W et al. MRI of cystic intracranial lesions. Radiology 1985; 155: 363–369.
36. Hubbard AM, Egelhoff JC. MR imaging of large hypothalamic hamartomas in two infants. AJNR 1989; 10: 1277.
37. Burton EM, Ball WS Jr, Crane K et al. Hamartomas of the tuber cinereum: comparison of CT and MR findings in 4 cases. AJNR 1989; 10: 497–502.
38. Arenzana-Suisdedos F, Barbey S, Virelizier JL. Histiocytosis X: purified (T6) cells from bone granulomata produce interleukin I and prostaglandin E2 in culture. J Clin Invest 1986; 77: 326–329.
39. Daningue JN, Wilson CB. Pituitary abscesses: report of 7 cases and review of the literature. J Neurosurg 1977; 46: 601–608.
40. Bossard D, Himed A, Badet C et al. MRI and CT in a case of pituitary abscess. J Neuroradiol 1992; 19: 139–144.
41. Gupta RK, Jena A, Sharma A et al. MR imaging of intracranial tuberculomas. J Comput Assist Tomogr 1988; 12: 280–285.
42. Berger SA, Edberg SC, David G. Infectious disease in the sella turcica. Rev Infect Dis 1986; 8: 747–755.
43. Martinez HR, Rangel-Guerra R, Elizondo G et al. MR imaging in neurocysticercosis: comparison with CT and anatomopathologic features. AJNR 1989; 10: 1011–1020.
44. Weisberg LA, Jacobs L. Clinical and computed tomography findings in intracranial sarcoidosis involving the juxtasellar region. Comput Radiol 1984; 8: 107–111.
45. Hayes WS, Sherman JL, Stern BJ et al. MR and CT evaluation of intracranial sarcoidosis. AJR 1987; 149: 1043–1049.
46. Kwan ESK, Wolpert SM, Hedges TR III et al. Tolosa–Hunt syndrome revisited: not necessarily a diagnosis of exclusion. AJNR 1987; 8: 1067–1072.
47. Yousem DM, Atlas SW, Grossman RI et al. MR imaging of Tolosa–Hunt syndrome. AJNR 1989; 10: 1181–1184.
48. Asa SL, Bilbao JM, Kovacs K et al. Lymphocytic hypophysitis of pregnancy resulting in hypopituitarism: a distinct clinicopathologic entity. Ann Intern Med 1981; 95: 166–169.
49. Goudie RB, Pinkerton PH. Anterior hypophysitis and Hashimoto's disease in a young woman. J Pathol Bacteriol 1962; 83: 584–558.

Surgery of pituitary adenomas

Michael Powell

This chapter sets out the surgical routes to the pituitary gland and gives an ordered approach to the removal of different types of pituitary adenomas. Its aim is to give the clinician who may not have seen operations on pituitary tumours some idea of what an operative procedure entails, as well as helping the surgeon, who may only see a handful of cases each year, to formulate ideas of surgical strategy.

SURGICAL ANATOMY

The pituitary gland is made of two parts. The anterior lobe, also known as the adenohypophysis, is a fibrous orange-pink glandular structure made up of secretory cells in a reticulin network, lying in front of the posterior lobe. This part, the neuropophysis, is an extension of the brain, a whitish-grey

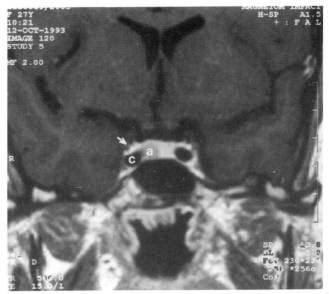

Fig. 6.1 Coronal MRI through the cavernous sinus and pituitary gland, with small adenoma (a) showing the third nerve (white arrow) and fourth nerve (black arrow) lateral to the carotid (c).

collection of nerve endings of the pituitary stalk. Neuroendocrinologists and anatomists recognize a third part, the pars intermedia, but it is unclear whether this tissue exists at all in man, or if it has been absorbed into the anterior pituitary tissue as a subgroup of the adrenocorticotrophic hormone (ACTH)-secreting cells. The two lobes lie in a depression in the skull base, the pituitary fossa, also known as the sella turcica (Turkish saddle) or simply the sella (cf. suprasellar—above the level of the upper limit of the sella). The sella is lined by a continuation of the dura mater, the membrane that surrounds the brain.

The floor and anterior wall of the sella are formed by the roof of the sphenoid air sinus, and the posterior wall by the clivus. The lateral borders are formed by the cavernous sinus—the complex venous structure that contains the carotid artery on its entry through the skull base through the foramen lacerum (it should be noted that the carotid arteries can encroach across the midline as seen in Fig. 6.2b, an important point if transsphenoidal surgery is considered)—and the three cranial nerves that control eye movements: the third, fourth and sixth (Fig. 6.1). The sinus is attached anteriorly to a rearward projection of the anterior fossa floor on either side of the midline, the anterior clinoid processes. At its posterior limit it is attached to the lateral tips of the clivus, also known as the posterior clinoid processes. The roof of the fossa is an incomplete fold of dura, the diaphragm sellae, through which the stalk passes. The stalk contains the fibres of the neuropophysis, which connect the posterior lobe to the supraoptic and para-

(a) (b)

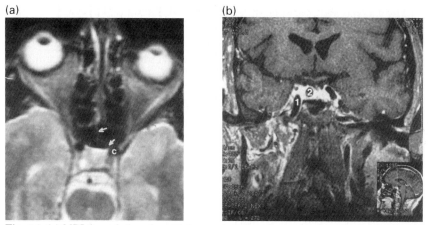

Fig. 6.2 (a) MRI through the sphenoid sinus and pituitary fossa, showing a deviated sphenoid septum (arrow) that starts anteriorly in the midline and lies over the left carotid (c) posteriorly. (**b**) Coronal MRI through a pituitary gland showing a right internal carotid that lies in the midline inferiorly (1) and in the midline in the middle of the gland (2).

ventricular nucleii of the hypothalamus, and the portal venous system, transmitting the hypothalamic peptides which control anterior lobe secretion, via the median eminence.

The fossa 'hangs' in the sphenoid air sinus, an air cavity extending from the anterior fossa floor to the clivus. Part or even occasionally all of the sinus may be incompletely pneumatized, and thus be made up of solid bone several millimetres thick. Usually the floor and anterior wall are 1 mm thick, with a variable number of septa which divide the sinus within. One of these is usually in the midline but may deviate markedly (Fig. 6.2a) or even be completely lateralized. Failure to appreciate the exact position of the septa can lead to severe risk of carotid damage in a transsphenoidal operation.

The sphenoid sinus is lined with nasal mucosa and is connected at its anteroinferior border by an opening, the sphenoid osteum, to the back of the nasal cavity near the vomer, the buttress of the nasal septum. Above the sinus lie the ethmoid air cells and anterior fossa floor of the cranial cavity.

Above the fossa itself lie the optic nerves and chiasm, separated from the hypothalamus and surrounded by cerebrospinal fluid (CSF). The optic nerves can either be short or long, so that the chiasm can lie close or far away from the optic foramen, known respectively as 'pre-fixed' or 'post-fixed'. A pre-fixed chiasm makes transcranial surgery extremely difficult by restricting access to the tumour mass which will lie behind this important and delicate structure, but symptoms will usually develop relatively early from early pressure on the back of the optic chiasm and tracts. Conversely, the post-fixed chiasm may allow a silent tumour to become huge, as the long intracranial portion of the nerves stretch around the edge of the tumour with little or no visual compromise.

The gland receives arterial blood from small branches of the carotid within the cavernous sinus, the superior hypophyseal and the meningohypophyseal arteries. It also receives the specialized venous supply from the portal system down the stalk. Venous drainage is to the cavernous sinus. The sinus has large interconnections across the front of the gland within the dura, the intercavernous sinuses. There are usually two, one above and one below, though they may form a complete lake. This may significantly interfere with the delicate exploration needed to remove a microadenoma, because of torrential venous bleeding.

CLINICAL PRESENTATION

Pituitary tumours may present in any of four general ways:

1. Endocrine dysfunction through either overproduction, as in acromegaly or Cushing's, or by underfunction as in Addisonian crises or secondary amenorrhoea
2. Mass effect on adjacent structures, usually the optic nerves and chiasm, but occasionally the third nerve with an attendant palsy, or even the third ventricle causing hydrocephalus
3. Headache, due to distortion of the dural structures at the skull base
4. Chance finding on radiological examination for some other reason.

Endocrine dysfunction is the most common, and headache and chance presentation infrequent.

SURGICAL AIMS

Each tumour poses a different problem with an individual surgical aim. Surgery can achieve:

1. Total tumour removal
2. Decompression of optic chiasm and adjacent structures
3. Tumour debulking
4. Tumour biopsy.

Hormone overproduction demands total tumour removal for an endocrine cure, although a temporary cure can be achieved by near-total removal in some cases. Improved vision can be achieved by quite modest tumour debulking, but the chance of a total surgical cure from any large lesion, particularly if it is suprasellar, is very small however successful the operation and surgery is only one part of the active treatment. Occasionally a large aggressive tumour expanding out of the fossa but without endocrine or compressive effects will simply require debulking prior to radiotherapy. Very infrequently the radiological diagnosis is uncertain, and a simple biopsy is required.

Table 6.1 The Hardy classification of pituitary adenomas (Hardy and Verzina, 1976)

Sella Turcica			Enclosed adenoma
Grade	0		Intact, with normal contour
	I		Intact, with focal bulging of floor
	II		Intact, enlarged fossa
	III	Invasive	⎰ Localized destruction
	IV		⎱ Diffuse destruction

Suprasellar			
Grade	A	⎫	⎧ To suprasellar cistern only
	B	⎬ Symmetrical	⎨ Recesses of third ventricle
	C	⎭	⎩ whole anterior third ventricle
	D	Asymmetrical	⎰ Intracranial extradural
	E		⎱ Extracranial extradural including lateral cavity sinus

CLASSIFICATION

Adenomas can be classified radiologically according to size; Table 6.1 illustrates the Hardy classification, which is generally used. It is simple and can aid surgical decision making. The radiological classification is of use as an aid to surgical strategy.

THE SURGICAL APPROACH

The approach can usually be decided on by tumour size alone.

Microadenomas (grades 0 and 1)

If surgery is considered the appropriate management, these tumours have to be approached via a transsphenoidal route to gain a direct view of the gland, as it is impossible to perform microdissection to separate tumour from the normal adenohypophysis transcranially. Should a transcranial procedure be carried out, the risk of total ablation of the gland is very high.

Whole sellar tumours (grades 2 and 3)

Transsphenoidal surgery is preferable to transcranial for these lesions, for the same reasons as in microadenomas. However, in very large macrosellar tumours, a significant decompression could be carried out transcranially, though it would be difficult to justify this approach, with its increased risks and less good results in relation to percentage of tumour clearance and preservation of endocrine function.

Tumours that extent laterally into the cavernous sinus (grade E) or even further into the subtemporal area are a very difficult problem as it is difficult to get into this area via either route. Transcranial approaches to the cavernous sinus are complicated and seldom justify the morbidity or complexity of an operative procedure in slow-growing, benign, pituitary adenomas. The third nerve is at risk from this approach. In a discussion at the pituitary adenoma session of the First International Skull Base Surgery Conference in Hanover in 1992, it was stated by Hardy that transsphenoidal dissection of the cavernous sinus is dangerous and should be avoided, but Fahlbusch held that it is possible for those with considerable experience of transsphenoidal surgery.

Suprasellar tumours (grades A, B, C and D)

Excellent results can be obtained from transsphenoidal decompression of these tumours, both from the chiasmal compression effects and endocrine preservation. This is particularly true of tumours which fit into categories A, B and C on the Hardy scale. For massive tumours, including the multilobulated (D and E), transsphenoidal surgery may be effective. If debulking is only partial, a second-stage operation will be necessary, often via a transcranial route. The capsule of these massive tumours may be very organized and full of collagen fibres, which makes transsphenoidal decompression and collapse of the tumour cavity impossible (Fig. 6.3).

Most modern pituitary surgeons agree that transcranial surgery should be a last resort. Even if it is necessary, a previous transsphenoidal decompression of limited type can be of great assistance in reducing tumour bulk, and in helping descent of the tumour dome into the operative field of a transcranial procedure.

Transsphenoidal surgery is not appropriate if the fossa is small or the diaphagm of the sella constricting (producing a 'cottage loaf' tumour), if the suprasellar component is causing compressive problems.

PRE-OPERATIVE WORKUP

Prior to pituitary surgery, every patient should have had:

1. Investigations:
   a. Endocrine assessment
   b. Eye field charting if the tumour is part suprasellar
   c. Adequate imaging to assess the fossa and its approaches, and to locate the tumour if small.

2. Cortisol cover: Prior to surgery all patients require cortisol cover, although an exception can be made for microadenomas secreting growth hormone (GH) or prolactin. In these tumours, it may be unnecessary if

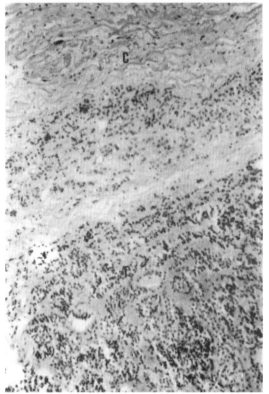

Fig. 6.3 Low-power photomicrograph of pituitary adenoma stained with haematoxylin and Van Geeson showing tumour (T) and collagen fibres of the capsule as wavy lines (C).

there is an almost intact normal gland. For reasons of safety, in the authors' unit even those patients with these small tumours receive the initial cortisol cover as part of the operative protocol, although they may not continue afterwards.

Hydrocortisone 100 mg is given with the anaesthetic pre-medication or on induction of the anaesthetic.

3. Antibiotic prophylaxis: the first dose is given at anaesthetic induction, followed by two further doses at 8 h intervals. A broad-spectrum antibiotic such as Cephaloridine 750 mg is recommended. Some experienced pituitary surgeons consider this unnecessary. (Landolt 86).

TRANSSPHENOIDAL SURGERY

Choice of route

There are four ways to approach and enter the sphenoid air sinus. The names of the surgeons who first promoted the approach are given in parentheses:

1. Transethmoidal (Angel-James)
2. Sublabial (Hardy/Cushing)
3. Direct transnasal (Griffith)
4. Septal endomucosal (Hirsch/Landolt).

Of these routes, the author prefers the last, believing it to be the best compromise between speed, safety and the least tissue disturbance.

The transethmoidal approach leaves a visible scar at the medial border of the eye with the bridge of the nose, and restricts a direct view of the upper part of the fossa. This can make surgery for the larger tumours particularly difficult, although its exponents would claim advantages of width of operative field and a short route.

Griffith's approach has the problem of muscosal bleeding during rectraction and removal of the septum at the vomer. Both this approach and the ethmoidal approach have a greater risk of loss of midline identification. If this occurs, there is a significant risk of straying into the carotid artery.

There is little to choose between the Hardy and Landolt routes except the latter is quicker and has minimal, if any, post-operative swelling and bruising. It is the Landholt approach with minor modifications that is discussed here.

EQUIPMENT

1. Operating microscope with zoom and viewing side arm for assistant
2. C arm fluoroscopy (image intensifier) or, if not available, peri-operative plain X-rays
3. Transsphenoidal intruments (see Fig. 6.4)
4. High-speed drill with long angled head.

Technique

Anaesthesia (see Ch. 7)

If the tumour has a suprasellar extension, a lumbar drain is inserted prior to the surgical approach, as will be discussed below.

Positioning

There are two positions for surgery: across the chest or at the head end of the table (Fig. 6.5). The author prefers the latter, with the operating table tilted head up. This position aids venous drainage and is more comfortable for the surgeon.

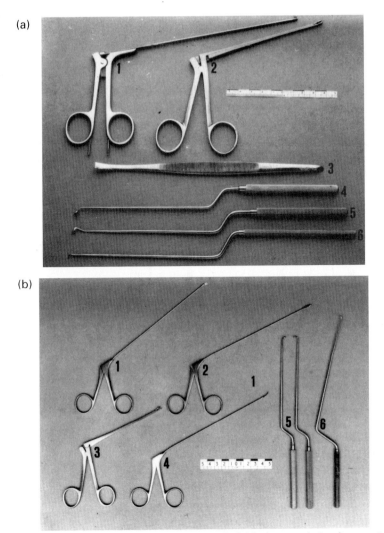

Fig. 6.4 Transsphenoidal intruments. (**a**) 1, Landholt bipolar coagulation forceps; 2, Angel James rongeurs; 3, dissector; 4, Hardy mirror; 5, Hardy dissector; 6, Fahlbusch dissector. (**b**) 1, Nicola scissors; 2, Fahlbusch cup rongeurs; 3, Angel James rongeurs; 4, Fahlbusch scissors; 5, Hardy ring curettes (2); 6, Fahlbusch spoon curette.

Preparation

The nose is prepared with an aqueous antiseptic and the right thigh with an alcohol antiseptic. Nasal vasoconstictors, either xylometazoline drops or Moffat's solution, should have been put in by the anaesthetist. These can significantly reduce nasal bleeding on average from 33 ml to 8 ml (unpublished data). Drapes are placed to leave the nose exposed and the

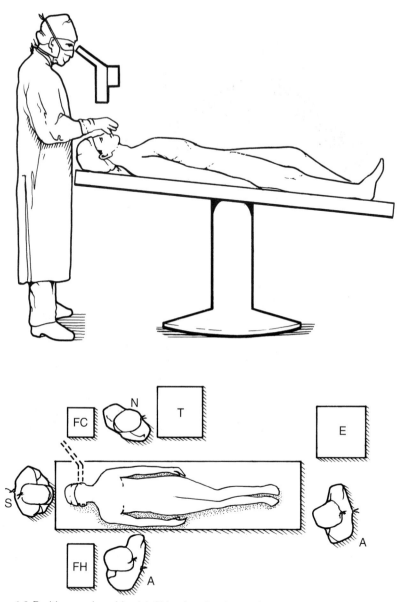

Fig. 6.5 Position on the table. (**a**) Side view showing patient, surgeon and microscope in schematic form. (**b**) Plan view showing S = surgeon, A = assistant, N = nurse with T = table and An = anaesthetist with E = equipment. The fluoroscope head (FH) and camera (FC) are also shown (microscope not shown).

thigh prepared for a fascia lata graft should it be necessary at the end of the tumour removal to reseal the fossa, in the event of a CSF leak.

Fascia is incorporated quickly into the fossa floor dura and sphenoid

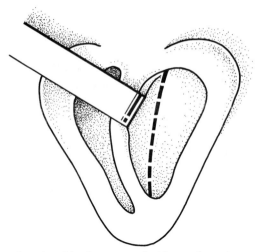

Fig. 6.6 Right nostril as viewed by the surgeon. Incision on the septum.

mucosa, forming a CSF-proof surface within 2–3 days. Our unit has not had a permanent CSF fistula in over 300 cases since fascia grafting was adopted.

Fascia has two advantages over abdominal fat, which is another frequently recommended and used sealing material. These are: firstly, ease of redissection if a second procedure is necessary and, secondly, less likelihood of a foul-smelling discharge as the excess fat putrifies, although the small abdominal scar used for a fat graft is cosmetically better than the small thigh incision for the fascia lata. Muscle, an old neurosurgical standby which is often used by more traditional surgeons, is totally unnecessary, as it is less effective than either fascia or fat, always putrifies and leaves a big scar.

Approach

The Landolt approach makes the first incision on the nasal septal mucosa in the right nostril, approximately 1 mm from its tip (Fig. 6.6). A tunnel is developed by blunt dissection between the nasal septal cartilage and the mucosa, using the Killian's retractors, starting with the shortest. The incision is carried inferiorly onto the premaxilla, and then swept laterally off the floor of the nose for 2–3 mm from the base of the septum. This is separated from the floor by gentle blunt dissection. If the nasal opening is very small, the incision can be carried on down into the inferior nares, with only a small external scar as the price (see Fig. 6.7).

The operating microscope is brought in and the mucosal tunnel further deepened until the junction between the cartilaginous and bony septum is seen (Fig. 6.8). The cartilage is separated from the bone, and the left-hand side of the nose entered under the septal mucosa. The mucosal tunnels are

(a) (b)

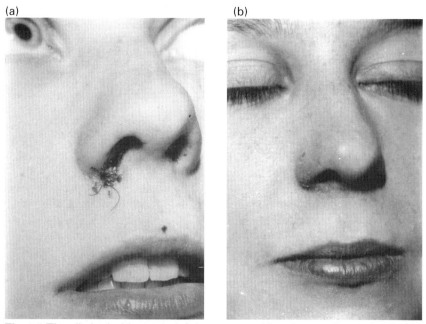

Fig. 6.7 The relieving incision on the inferior nares seen (**a**) on the second post-operative day and (**b**) invisible at 2 months.

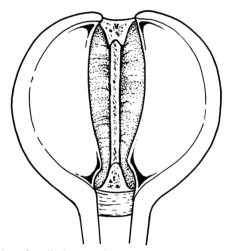

Fig. 6.8 At the junction of cartilaginous and bony septum.

further deepened on either side until the vomer is encountered at the roof of the nose. It is helpful to remove the bony septum with a small pituitary rongeur. The position of the rectractor should be checked at regular intervals with X-ray screening (Fig. 6.9).

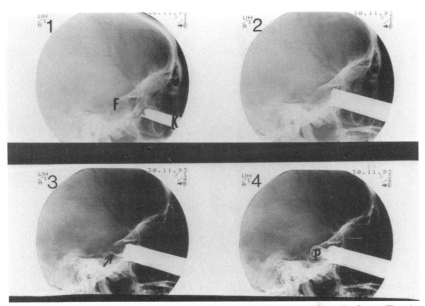

Fig. 6.9 Lateral skull fluoroscopy screening showing (**1**) the approach to the fossa (F) using Killians retractor (K); (**2**) the Landholt retractor in position; (**3**) the fossa emptied and the floor outlined with contrast, shown as a white line (arrow); and (**4**) the fossa filled with cottonoid patties soaked in contrast (P).

At the vomer the definitive Landolt or Hardy rectractor (Fig. 6.10) is placed and the space opened. Each has its advantges, the former being slimmer and more delicate, but they are essentially the same, both being modifications of the original Cushing design. A small mucosal artery is seen arising from the sphenoid approximately 4 mm from the midline (Fig. 6.11). It may require bipolar coagulation. Its origin should sit at or near the tip of the inferior blade of the retractor. If it does not, the retractor position is too low. The vomer and sphenoid rostrum are drilled away with the high-speed drill using a cutting burr and the sphenoid air sinus entered. The pituitary fossa is now seen from below. The hole into the sinus can be extended with ethmoid punches (2 mm angled up and down being useful) to obtain the best view of the fossa (Fig. 6.12).

The mucosa of the sinus is removed along with any sphenoidal septum to get the best view of the front of the fossa. It is not essential to remove every fragment of mucosa, despite a widely held surgical misconception that mucoceles will occur if not done. The mucosal blood supply comes through the bone and a small venous ooze develops following mucosal stripping. This soon settles down without intervention.

The superior and inferior borders of the fossa can now be defined on

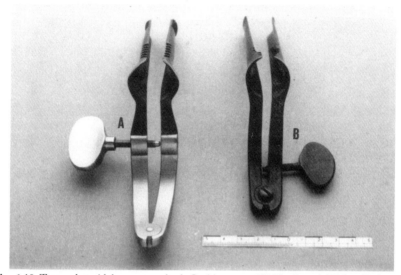

Fig. 6.10 Transsphenoidal retractors, both Cushing type: (**A**) Hardy and (**B**) Landholt.

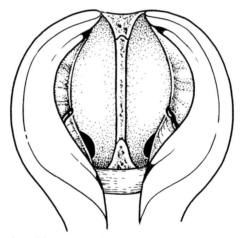

Fig. 6.11 At the junction of the vomer and anterior wall of the sphenoid fossa.

fluoroscopy. Particular attention *must* be paid to the exact position of the septum in relation to the carotids, for the reasons previously mentioned. The bone of the fossa is now carefully drilled away using the diamond burr (Fig. 6.13). This method, though slower than using dental chisels, is more controlled, and is therefore safer. With the burr, one never 'plunges' into the carotid, as the author has witnessed when watching the chisel method being demonstrated. Furthermore, the diamond burr has the advantage of being haemostatic to bone, thus minimizing bleeding at an important stage.

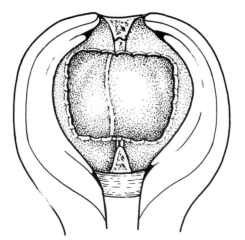

Fig. 6.12 After opening of the anterior pituitary fossa wall.

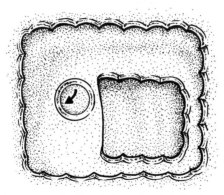

Fig. 6.13 Bone of the fossa opened with orih (arrow) on left. Further opening achieved with punches exposing dura (shown on right).

In large tumours the floor of the fossa is often so thinned by the tumour pressure that either of these methods is unecessary, as the bone flakes incompletely cover the fossa floor and may be simply lifted off.

The hole into the fossa can be widened with 1 and 2 mm ethmoid punches, carefully protecting the dura to keep it intact. The opening is taken laterally to the cavernous sinus which appears as a purplish tinge in the dura, and superiorly to the junction of the anterior fossa floor. Inferiorly, the limits may be the purplish intercavernous sinus or where the anterior wall turns back to become the floor.

The dura can now be opened. If a large intercavernous sinus lies in the way, unipolar coagulation over the fossa surface will control this (Laws, personal comunication). Sharp dissection using either an '11' blade on the cranked Hardy pituitary scalpel or pituitary microscissors is recommended for opening the dura, as it is more controlled than the unipolar cutting wand sometimes used. The incision is taken diagonally from side to side, forming a diagonal cross. The limits are the sinuses, which should be avoided as they bleed profusely if entered. Dural bleeding can be controlled by bipolar coagulation, pressure from small patties or gelatine sponge pledgets. Some surgeons recommend excising dura because of the risk of dural invasion.

The gland and tumour can now be inspected. The procedure differs from this point depending on the size of the tumour and operative aim.

Small (usually hormone overproduction) tumours. Small tumours have to be found. This may seem obvious, and it is usually straightforward. However, 2–4 mm microadenomas can be extremely challenging.

The normal gland is a fibrous pink-orange, whereas a tumour is soft and creamy white or pale grey, and seldom has a fibrous stroma, as adenomas do not have a reticulin network. However, some bromocriptine pre-treated prolactinomas can be very fibrotic. The author has not found the descriptions of the likely positions of the various types of secreting adenomas, as given by Hardy, particularly useful.

Once found, the tumour is dissected from the normal gland, if possible shaving off the normal gland adjacent to it, using Hardy and Fahlbusch microdissectors, Hardy ring curettes and the various microscissors. The gland functions perfectly well on 20% of normal volume, so a reasonable fringe can be taken. The tumour bed can be filled with an absolute alcohol-soaked patty or gelfoam plug in an attempt to kill any residual tumour, although Hardy has been heard to comment that alcohol should be reserved for the surgeon after the operation, not for the patient during it. There is no evidence that the use of alcohol improves the endocrine outcome.

If the tumour cannot be found (this most commonly occurs in Cushing's tumours) and there has been localizing help from either pre-operative sinus sampling or radiology, the surgeon can remove the half of the lobe that the tumour 'should' be in, but must realize that the chances of cure are less high than if an adenoma is found. If an endocrine cure is not effected, a second procedure can be offered within a few days to remove the remaining anterior lobe. If there is no localizing help, the surgeon has either to guess and remove the half thought to be the most suspicious of tumour, or remove the whole lobe. In either case the strategy should be discussed carefully with the patient before the first operation.

Sadly, even removing the whole gland may not always effect a cure. Either the diagnosis of a pituitary-dependent disease is wrong, or cell nests of tumour along the stalk up to the median eminence, and beyond the reach of transsphenoidal surgery, continue to produce their hormone-releasing effect.

Large sella tumours. The dissection is usually simpler than in microadenomas, as there is no problem in finding the tumour. However, it is more difficult to be certain of complete tumour removal, if the aim is to effect an endocrine cure. Mirrors are of significant use at this point to study the cavernous sinus wall for tumour remnants. Small extensions into the cavernous sinus can be very difficult to find, although a high intrasellar pressure, measured at the time of entry into the gland, is a method used by some surgeons at the time of the dissection to identify this problem. Again, tumour removal is effected using ring curettes, dissectors and rongeurs. Filmy remnants of the tumour are often found once the last bulk of the tumour is removed, and must be removed. Resecting the normal gland adjacent to the adenoma is usually impossible, hence the endocrine results of surgery are less good (see Ch. 8).

Suprasellar tumours. The fossa is emptied of tumour first. The suprasellar portion of the tumour will be seen pulsating with respiration and pulse at the superior border of the fossa. This can be brought down safety into the operative field by injection of saline into the lumbar drain. This is carried out slowly, in 5 ml aliquots, by the anaesthetist, whilst blood pressure and pulse are carefully monitored. Usually the dome gently descends, aided by being gently broken up by a Hardy dissector. The capsule, formed by the normal residual gland (flattened like 'strudel dough' according to Fahlbusch) and the arachnoid, is seen as a thin grey-purple semi-transluscent structure, and is usually quite easy to distinguish and thus can be kept intact.

Technical details

Haemostasis

Pituitary tumours are not as a rule vascular. Once the tumour is out, the small venous ooze is controlled by gentle patty pressure, which if troublesome can be replaced by gelatine sponge or similar aid to coagulation. Similarly, sinus bleeding can be stopped in the same way. If there is little or no ooze, nothing needs to placed in the fossa or in the dural defect. Alternatively, some surgeons prefer to cover the defect with a sheet of gelatin sponge.

CSF leaks

These are usually small and occur from a fold of arachnoid at the superior part of the anterior wall of the gland. They may sometimes be stoped by 'tacking' the dura to the arachnoid with bipolar coagulation. If this fails or the leak is profuse, then a patch of fascia lata from the thigh placed over the dural defect will form a perfect seal. A lumbar drain, if not already in place, should be set, draining at bed height to create zero intracranial pressure. The patient is nursed flat for 2–3 days.

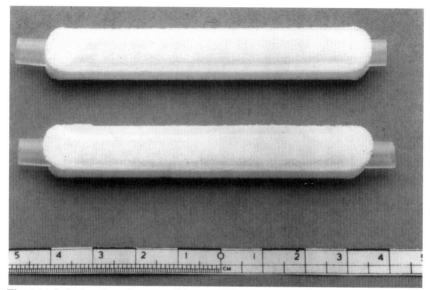

Fig. 6.14 Dehydrated nasal sponges (Merocet, USA).

Closure

The rectractor is removed, the cartilaginous septum pushed back into position, and the mucosa repaired with two or three catgut sutures. Catgut is used because it dissolves quickly, whilst more modern suture material lasts for a long time and often disturbs the patient by hanging from their nose for weeks. Dehydrated sponges (Fig. 6.14) are placed into the nostrils and dampened with saline. These swell and gently tamponade the operated area.

Reoperations

Repeat transsphenoidal surgery can be very difficult. Loss of the normal landmarks makes it easy to lose the midline and stray into the cavernous sinus or carotids. If at all possible, the original operation note should be studied, to find out what was done, and which route and which packing material were used. The best-quality radiology should be obtained, including computed tomography (CT), if there is any question about bony landmarks. CT gives much better information about residual bony septa than magnetic resonance imaging (MRI), although the best modern MRI can give good information. On older machines this detail is completely lost.

The approach is essentially the same. It often helps to use a different approach from the original, especially if one was not the first surgeon, as some of the normal landmarks may have remained untouched. A slow technique, checking frequently with fluoroscopy, is recommended. If care is used, and the tissues still remain, the correct operative plains can be re-established. This is particularly true along the remnants of the bony septum, where careful blunt dissection with the Hardy dissector is very helpful.

At the sphenoid air sinus, the packing material must be stripped out, and the anterior wall remnants of the fossa identified. Again, the use of the fluoroscope is essential. The fossa wall has a surprising ability to regenerate, and may be almost complete. It is usually obvious why an original operation for microadenoma failed, almost always because of incomplete exposure of the front of the gland, which means that some 'normal' unoperated tissue remains to be explored.

For larger tumours or regrowth, the key to success is getting into the tumour bulk. Success may be thwarted by extensive post-operative fibrous septa that block the dissection. In this case a further transcranial procedure will be inevitable.

Coping with disasters

There are two events which constitute a disaster; both occur because of loss of the landmarks to the fossa. The least infrequent is carotid damage, which this author has not caused although has managed the consequences.

If the carotid is entered, the procedure comes to a rapid halt whilst the worried surgeon gets control with packing. This is usually successful in the short term and the patient is allowed to recover normally. However, it is essential to perform carotid angiography, as there may well be a false aneurysm, as can be seen in Figure 6.15(a) on MRI (T1-weighted image) and Figure 6.15(b) on angiography. This aneurysm, if untreated, may lead to torrential arterial bleeding, as it did in this case, at about 10 days from surgery. In the night this may be fatal, as the patient can exsanguinate before the startled staff can gain control by direct carotid pressure. The false aneurysm must be obliterated, either angiographically with coils or balloons, or by surgical exclusion, with clipping above and below the cavernous carotid.

The second disaster comes from missing the fossa altogether, and opening the clivus behind. As reported in the popular press but never seen by this author, biopsy of the pons, lying behind, has serious consequences to the patient. For the novice and expert alike, checking the position of the fossa radiographically is of vital importance prior to opening.

TRANSCRANIAL SURGERY

Inevitably, the surgeon will have to carry out transcranial surgery on occasion. This only occurs in our unit if the transsphenoidal procedure has been a failure. There are two routes to choose from, both with their firm

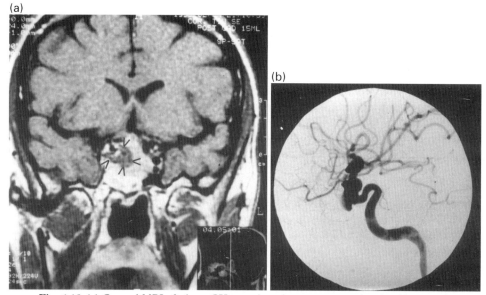

Fig. 6.15 (**a**) Coronal MRI of a large GH-secreting adenoma compressing the chiasm, and a traumatic post-operative aneurysm extending into the fossa. (**b**) Angiogram of **a**.

adherents: the subfrontal and the pterional. These two options are, in essence, only different by a few millimetres on the anterior fossa floor, the key being in both that the anterior bone cut in the craniotomy be as close to the fossa floor as possible, which will then minimize frontal lobe rectraction.

Pre-operative investigations

As for transsphenoidal surgery, although MRI or very good-quality CT is essential.

Careful study of the pre-operative MRI will tell the surgeon if the chiasm is pre-fixed, in which case the more anterior subfrontal route may be preferable as it gives the surgeon the option of opening the lamina terminalis above the chiasm in order to get to the dome of the tumour. The MRI will also give valuable information about the carotids, making pre-operative angiography redundant. The size and position of the frontal air sinuses must also be studied from the scans, which if large may be opened in the subfrontal approach. If the pterional route is adopted, a post-chiasmal mass can be debulked in the small space between the third nerve and the back of the supraclinoid carotid. This gap is, however, challengingly small.

Pre-operative loading with high-dose steroids is given (Dexamethasone 4 mg q.i.d.) for brain proctection. Prophylactic antibiotics are given with anaesthetic induction. There is probably little value is giving anti-convulsants, although it is often done.

Anaesthesia and positioning

The patient is anaesthetized and placed supine on the table. Head-up tilt is helpful. The skin is prepared in the preferred way—in this unit with Hibitane in 70% alcohol.

Approach

A bicoronal incision gives the best cosmetic result and the amount of hair shaved is minimal, if any. In fact, most frontal incisions heal almost invisibly, even if they extend onto the forehead.

With the skin turned down, the pericranium is opened and burr holes placed for the craniotomy. In a young patient this may only require a single one hidden under the temporalis muscle, but in the elderly, where the dura is both thin and adherent, multiple holes are recommended. If the frontal air sinus is opened, the mucosa is stripped out of the bone flap, and obliteration of the sinus planned for the end stages of the procedure, usually by swinging a flap of pericranium over the defect in the supraorbital bone and gluing it into position with human fibrin glue.

The dura is opened over the anterior fossa floor and the brain gently elevated. The floor is followed back to the planum sphenoidale—the flat area that lies between the optic foramina—where the right optic nerve will be seen, usually pushed fowards by the tumour. A fold of arachnoid usually protects the frontal lobe from the tumour surface. The brain is separated here and the tumour wall further exposed between the two nerves, although the left optic nerve is usually seen rather later on in the procedure. The tumour can now be entered, using bipolar coagulation and sharp dissection of the capsule. Once access is made, the interior is gutted, allowing the capsule to be peeled from the optic nerves and hypothalamus using a combination of sharp and blunt dissection.

Behind the capsule, the stalk will be seen running into the remnants of the normal gland, a disc on the capsule surface. The remainder of the chiasm will also be seen medial to the carotids and their bifurcation into middle and anterior cerebral arteries.

Residual fragments are dissected away with sharp dissection and haemostasis achieved, usually with oxidized cellulose sheets (Surgicel) to the fossa bed, for, as previously stated, bleeding is seldom a major problem once the bulk of the tumour is removed. The retraction is removed and the skull and its membranes reconstituted according to standard practice.

Complications

The major difficulty experienced by the surgeon new to skull base work is failure to get low enough to obtain sufficient view of the tumour. The approach along the anterior fossa floor is essential, otherwise needless and damaging frontal lobe retraction is necessary.

Failure to appreciate the position of the chiasm may also lead to the surgeon arriving at the chiasm with little view of the tumour behind. There are a number of choices at this point. The approach behind the carotid is a possibility, as mentioned, although there is not much space, especially if the tumour bleeds. Removal of the planum sphenoidale and an approach creating space below the chiasm by bone removal is also suggested as a possibility (Symon, personal communication). The recommended approach by Samii is through the lamina terminalis, above the chiasm and through the third ventricle. Sacrifice of an optic nerve is another option which may be worth considering if the function in one eye is very severely compromised.

FURTHER READING

Fahlbusch R, Honneger J, Buchfelder M. Surgical management of acromegaly. Endocrinol Metab Clin North Am 1992; 21: 669–692.

Griffith HB, Veerapen R. A direct transnasal approach to the sphenoid sinus. J Neurosurg 1987; 66: 185.

Hardy J, Verzina JL. Transsphenoidal neurosurgery of intracranial neoplasm. In: Thompson RA, Green JR (eds) Advances in neurology. New York: Raven Press, 1976; pp 261–274 (updated at the International Pituitary Conference, Zurich, 1987).

Hardy J. Atlas of transsphenoidal microsurgery in pituitary tumours. New York: Igaku-Shoin, 1991.

Landolt A, Gammert Ch. Transsphenoidal surgery for pituitary adenomas. Tuttlingen, Germany: Aesculap, 1986. (This beautifully illustrated sales brochure is the best English description of the Landolt–Hirsch technique, although Landolt also describes the technique elsewhere in German.)

Symon L, Jakubowski J. Transcranial management of pituitary adenomas with suprasellar extension. J Neurol Neurosurg Psychiatry 1979; 42: 123–133.

Tindall GT, Barrow DL. Disorders of the pituitary (chapter on pituitary surgery). St Louis: Mosby, 1986; pp 349–400.

Anaesthesia for pituitary surgery

CHAPTER
7

Nicholas Hirsch, Doreen Jewkes

Pre-operative assessment
Pre-medication
Monitoring
Induction and maintenance of anaesthesia
Lumbar drainage
Post-operative care

Anaesthesia for pituitary surgery, whether performed via an anterior crani-otomy or via the transsphenoidal route, requires careful pre-operative assess-ment and meticulous peri- and post-operative management using principles common to all intracranial procedures.

Endocrinologically inactive pituitary tumours usually present when they become large enough to produce chiasmal compression with or without compression syndromes of the cavernous sinus or suprachiasmal structures. It is important for the anaesthetist to be aware that raised intracranial pressure may be present either due to the large size of the tumour or through obstruction of CSF outflow at the third ventricle causing hydrocephalus (see Ch. 4).

Hypersecretion of active hormones by a pituitary tumour will give rise to the typical syndromes as described in Chapter 3, although on occasion even these tumours may be large enough to cause mass effect, typically prolactinomas in the male, infrequently growth hormone (GH)-secreting tumours and, even rarer, giant Cushing's tumours.

141

PRE-OPERATIVE ASSESSMENT

Patients should have had a general medical asseement and, in addition, be assessed for the feature of raised intracranial presure (papilloedema, drowsiness, etc.). Patients with Cushing's disease or acromegaly must be fully assessed for coexisting systemic conditions.

Cushing's disease

Hypertension due to increased renin–angiotensin activity and increased blood volume is present in 85% of these patients. It should be adequately treated pre-operatively. Diabetes mellitus is present in 60% of these patients and control of blood glucose is essential before surgery. Renal function must also be assessed as calculi are common in this group. High circulating levels of glucocorticoids are immunosuppressive and coexisting infection, if present, must be brought under control.

Acromegaly

GH hypersecretion not only affects the extremities but also results in soft tissue swelling of the mouth, tongue and laryngeal cartilages. Careful assessment of the airway using the Mallampati criteria should be performed in an attempt to predict difficult tracheal intubation. Obstructive sleep apnoea is more common in acromegalic patients and a history of loud snoring, apnoeic periods during sleep and daytime hypersomnolescence should alert the anaesthetist to this possibility.

Hypertension occurs in 30% of patients, but in contrast to Cushing's disease is mild and easy to control. Cardiomegaly is routinely found and may be associated with a reduced left ventricular ejection fraction. Glucose intolerance is common and frank diabetes is present in 25% of patients. It requires control pre-operatively. Thyroid enlargement (often nodular) may be associated although under-functon is unusual.

Prolactinomas

Patients with these pituitary tumours usually present with menstrual disorders or infertility, and are usually without systemic disorders relevant to the anaesthetist.

PRE-MEDICATION

Traditionally sedative pre-medication is withheld for patients undergoing neurosurgical procedures. In cases where anxiolysis is deemed necessary, a small dose of benzodiazepine is appropriate. It is essential to continue antihypertensive therapy up to the time of surgery. Additional steroid cover should be given to patients undergoing surgery for Cushing's disease. Patients with severe diabetes should be managed with an insulin infusion. Pituitary surgery via a frontal craniotomy involves a degree of frontal lobe retraction with the attendant risk of post-operative seizures. Some surgeons prefer, therefore, to institute anticonvulsant prophylaxis in the pre-operative period, in which case levels should be checked.

MONITORING

Before induction, the patient should be monitored with ECG (modified CM_5 configuration), non-invasive blood pressure and oxygen saturation. After induction, direct arterial blood pressure measurement via a radial artery is used. A large-bore intravenous cannula should be used for venous access.

INDUCTION AND MAINTENANCE OF ANAESTHESIA

Anaesthesia is induced with thiopentone 5–7 mg/kg and fentanyl 1–2 μg/kg. Muscle relaxation prior to tracheal intubation is effected using a non-depolarizing neuromuscular blocking agent (e.g. atracurium). Acromegalic patients may be difficult to intubate and may require an awake fibre-optic intubation. Whichever method of endotracheal intubation is used, a nylon-reinforced tracheal tube should be used to prevent kinking intra-operatively. If the procedure is to be carried out transsphenoidally, a throat pack is inserted to prevent excessive accumulation of blood in the nasopharynx and the stomach. In addition, a vasoconstricting agent (eg a xylometazoline solution or a solution of cocaine 8% in bicarbonate) is introduced into each nostril; this mixture produces a relatively blood-free operative site. Following intubation, the patient should be mechanically ventilated to an end-tidal carbon dioxide tension of 4 kPa. The patient should continue to be moderately hyperventilated. Excessive hypocarbia should be avoided as the loss of brain bulk will make any suprasellar extension less accessible from below. Maintenance of anaesthesia is with additional short-acting opioid drugs (e.g. fentanyl and alfentanil), and with low concentrations of an inhalational anaesthetic agent. Isoflurane, with its rapid recovery profile, is the agent of choice.

Intra-operative hypertension should be treated with beta-blockade (e.g. labetalol) or with hydralazine.

At the end of the procedure, neuromuscular blockade is reversed and, following the return of sponaneous ventilation, the patient is extubated following removal of the throat pack. In the case of transsphenoidal surgery, this should only be carried out when the laryngeal reflexes have returned, so as to decrease the risk of pulmonary aspiration of blood which has pooled in the nasopharynx.

LUMBAR DRAINAGE

If the patient has a significant suprasellar extension, a lumbar drain is often required. This is inserted after the patient has been anaesthetized. In the lateral position, a 16G catheter is inserted at the L3–4 interspace using a Tuohy needle. After piercing the dura, 10 cm of the catheter are introduced in a cephalad direction into the subarachnoid space. Subsequent introduction of 10 ml aliquots of saline into this space will, during trans-sphenoidal surgery, produce prolapse of the suprasellar portion of the tumour into the operative field in the majority of cases. The catheter may also be left in place at the end of the procedure as a cerebrospinal fluid (CSF) drain, to control a CSF leak if the dura has been breached during the procedure (see breach of the dura, Chapter 6).

POST-OPERATIVE CARE

This consists of careful airway management, the provision of adequate post-operative analgesia, appropriate fluid replacement and careful monitoring of the development of diabetes insipidus (as described earlier).

Maintenance of a clear airway requires diligence; the presence of blood in the naso- and oropharynx, nasal packs and a predisposition of the acromegalic patient to obstruct the airway all tend to compromise airway patency. The patient should therefore be kept under close observation until fully awake.

Analgesia is usually provided by intramuscular codeine phosphate 45–60 mg every 2–4 h.

Normal saline is the maintenance fluid of choice in the post-operative period. If diabetes insipidus does occur, meticulous fluid balance must be maintained (see Chapter 8).

Post-operative management

Michael Powell,
Stafford Lightman

This chapter sets out the two stages of post-pituitary surgery management:

1. Immediate, both for functioning adenomas and for those tumours that cause symptoms through mass effect
2. The long-term management considering both endocrine function and the management of residual tumour causing either endocrine or mass symptoms.

A guide to the selection of patients in whom the aims of surgery are incompletely achieved and who may benefit either from further surgery or radiotherapy will be outlined, as well as the decision process for frequency of follow-up. The benefits of multidisciplinary pituitary clinics will be discussed.

As the majority of patients will have undergone transsphenoidal surgery, these patients will be considered in greater detail, although many of the same principles apply to those who have undergone craniotomy, including making post-operative testing of visual fields and acuity mandatory.

IMMEDIATE

Transsphenoidal surgery

General considerations

In general patients do not have many problems following transsphenoidal surgery. Patients need to be protected against the effects of pituitary dysfunction caused by the surgery, i.e. from failure of anterior lobe corticotrophs to secrete adrenocorticotrophic hormone (ACTH) in response to stress, resulting in the need for cortisol replacement, and from posterior lobe damage resulting in abnormalities of vasopressin (ADH) secretion which may lead to inappropriate oversecretion (SIADH) but much more commonly diabetes insipidus (DI) and the loss of large volumes of dilute urine.

Patients seldom need intensive nursing on a one-to-one basis, unless there are coexistent medical problems. Therefore, few patients need to go to an intensive care unit, and once they have awoken from the anaesthetic on a recovery unit may return to their normal bed on the ward. Nursing observations should include 4-hourly blood pressure, pulse and temperature and a fluid balance chart, but need not include neurological observations unless the patient had a macroadenoma involving vision and the hypothalamus.

Pain, fluid replacement and fluid balance

Simple analgesia is usually sufficient for post-operative pain, as it is not a particularly painful form of surgery. Most patients start oral fluids within a few hours, so intravenous fluids can be discontinued early, usually within the first 24 h. One litre of dextrose saline in 12 h is sufficient intravenous replacement. Urine output and specific gravity are both measured to identify in the early stages the development of DI, should it occur.

Post-operatively, DI usually occurs by the end of the first 24 h and should be suspected if the patient is producing more than a litre of dilute urine in 12 h, and the serum sodium is above 143 mmol/l. Urinary flow rates alone are insufficient evidence for the diagnosis of DI, as delayed excretion of the fluid load given during the operation, the use of osmotic diuretics and even corticosteroid-induced hyperglycaemia can all lead to polyuria. The diagnosis must be based on a combination of increased plasma osmolarity (>300 mosmol/kg), hypotonic urine (<300 mosmol/kg) and a urine flow rate of >2ml/kg per hour. This is in the absence of renal failure, hyperglycaemia and the use of osmotic diuretics.

If the patient is conscious and has a normal thirst mechanism, it is always safer to allow free access to fluid if there is any doubt about the diagnosis of DI, as over-enthusiastic use of DDAVP may lead to hyponatraemia, with its attendant problems of confusion, epileptic fits and ultimately coma and death, whereas a high urine output is an inconvenience to the patient, but not intrinsically dangerous.

It should be noted that many patients feel thirsty, because of mouth breathing, when nasal packs are in place in the early post-operative period. This should not be interpreted as a sign of DI without objective evidence. As the nasal tampons may be safely removed at 24 h, interpreting the early post-operative will to drink as DI should be resisted.

Some patients have borderline results suggesting partial DI. So long as they have a normal thirst mechanism, it is usually safer to resist DDAVP administration, avoiding the risk of overhydration. Most borderline cases recover normal posterior lobe function within a few days. Comatose patients and those showing no thirst response are at particular risk from both over- and underhydration. In these patients, treatment with desmopressin should only be repeated if polyuria recurs. In all at-risk patients plasma sodium should be monitored daily, until normal water balance has been clearly reestablished.

Nasal packs/tampons

These may be removed on the first post-operative day, for which mild sedation and analgesia are sometimes needed. Removed this early, clot does not organize around the tampons, which may be removed with minimal discomfort. There seems little justification for leaving the packs in from 3 up to 10 days, as is practised in some centres, at which time very heavy sedation and analgesia must be administered prior to removal. The self-dissolving sutures used do not need removal, but if a suture has been used to close a relieving incision in the inferior nares it must be removed. The scar left is shown in Figure 6.7.

Antibiotic prophylaxis

There is little logic applied to this subject. Although the majority of units use some form of prophylaxis, both Landolt and Fahlbusch, with two of the biggest series in the world, use none and claim no problems. In our unit, as in the majority of surgical units of every speciality in Britain, there is a policy for all patients undergoing surgery of any type to receive antibiotics. We use a three-dose regime using Cefuroxime 750 mg i.v., starting at induction of anaesthesia and continuing for two further doses at 8 and 16 h. There seems little need to employ the 3, 5 and even 10-day regimes used in some units, as this will promote the colonization of the nose with resistant organisms.

Complications

In experienced hands, complications are relatively rare. In a series of 67 consecutive patients undergoing surgery for large tumours causing visual problems, no mortality and only 14 events that were considered com-plications were reported. Of these 5 were transient CSF leaks which were easily dealt with as described below, none being prolonged. Four patients had transient diabetes insipidus, which settled in all but one case within the "in patient" peri-operative period, the single case persisting for 3 months. A single patient suffered a non fatal cardiopulmonary event and another elderly patient a period of temporary post operative confusion.

The most serious complications were in 3 patients who had post-operative haematomas within the tumour bed on post operative scanning. In one 70 year old woman, this caused a worsening of vision, although her vision improved compared to her initial pre-operative assessment some months later, following a second transsphenoidal procedure.

The management of the problems that can occur at transsphenoidal surgery are discussed below.

Cerebrospinal fluid leaks

These are fortunately infrequent. If a leak does occur during the procedure, it may be contained with a lumbar drain and a fascia graft, as is discussed in the Chapter 5. These will have been placed at the end of the operative procedure. The drain should be set at the height of the patient's head, and allows the assimilation of the fascia graft during the first 48 h. The patient is nursed head up. The drain should not produce more than 20 ml per hour. It may be switched off after the second day, and removed 12–24 h later, assuming that the leak does not redevelop.

If a leak develops after the procedure following the return to the ward, it may well settle with a lumbar drain alone, as the site of the leak was not recognized at the time of surgery and should therefore be very small.

In two patients in the author's series, blood in the cerebrospinal fluid (CSF) led to mild hydrocephalus sufficient to halt the patients' progress. Both required a ventriculoperitoneal shunt. However, the development of this complication is extremely rare.

Cortisol replacement

It is safest to assume that all patients will require replacement. All will have been given hydrocortisone 100 mg. i.v. with induction. Following surgery hydrocortisone may be tailed down to replacement levels within a few days. In our unit we give 50 mg b.d. for the first post-operative day, 25 mg. b.d. on the second, and reduce to 20 mg a.m. and 10 mg p.m. on the third. Patients usually leave hospital on this dose, although it is slightly above.the normal replacement of 15 mg a.m. and 5 mg p.m. Consequently, most patients will complain of some weight gain at the first follow-up 6 weeks later, but will be safe during this period from the dangers of low plasma cortisol. Most patients require their second dose at the end of the working day rather than at bedtime, when cortisol requirements are at their lowest. The p.m. dose should normally be given between 5 p.m. and 6 p.m.

Patients who have undergone transsphenoidal resection for prolactin or growth hormone-secreting microadenomas rarely have need for long-term replacement. If at least 20% of the normal gland has been left behind, the patient can be safely weaned off hydrocortisone during the first few days, without the risk of having suppressed the normal corticotrophs in the few days on steroid replacement. This does not apply to patients with successfully treated Cushing's tumours in whom the normal corticotrophs are heavily suppressed and who will usually need replacement for some weeks or even months.

Histopathological analysis

These results are eagerly awaited by most patients, regardless of any reassurance given to them that these tumours are virtually never malignant, and that there were no signs of features suggesting otherwise. The immunocytochemical results seldom alter management strategies, although they are of interest. Frequently, 'non-functioning' tumours do exhibit some hormone-containing granules within the cytoplasm, which contain either hormone precursors, luteinizing hormone (LH), or follicle-stimulating hormone (FSH) or non-secreted hormone such as ACTH. The significance of these changes is uncertain. Malignant change, very rarely encountered, or significant mitotic activity would lead to an early referral for radiotherapy.

Length of stay

Once the patient is up and mobile, with stable fluid balance and hormone replacement, there is little that needs to keep them in hospital. In the UK most patients may leave within 4 or 5 days, whereas in the USA financial considerations imposed by diagnosis-related group management causes most patients, if well, to be discharged from hospital within 48–72.

In our unit, all patients have the function for which they underwent the operation checked prior to discharge. Thus, patients with acromegaly undergo a glucose challenge with GH measurement, those with prolactinomas a single prolactin estimation, and Cushing's patients a fasting early-morning cortisol 24 h after temporarily stopping cortisol replacement. These tests may delay the early discharge of the patient, but do allow a useful, early estimation of the endocrine success of the procedure which will be available at the first review. Patients with eye field loss should have the first estimation of their eye fields at discharge.

Hyponatraemia

This complication of transsphenoidal surgery has already been mentioned in relation to over-enthusiastic use of DDAVP. However, it may occur spontaneously as part of the syndrome of inappropriate secretion of ADH

(SIADH) caused by a non-specific release of ADH from degenerating posterior pituitary neurosecretory terminals. This is usually transitory and rarely lasts more than a week to 14 days. This is another reason why a regular check on electrolytes should be made, and if a patient who has otherwise done well from the surgery feels unwell in a non-specific way at the time of discharge, check again! The condition is managed by fluid restriction. The clinical condition lags behind the electrolyte recovery, so the patient may continue confused with normal plasma sodium.

Special considerations

Acromegaly. Most acromegalic patients undergo substantial change within the first few days of surgery if cured. Sweating stops, the hands and feet shrink and the face slims down. Many of these changes can occur in the pre-operatively floridly acromegalic even if the patient is not completely cured.

Prolactinomas. The majority of operations carried out in our unit are on patients who are either resistant to or intolerant to bromocriptine and other dopamine agonists. Most have secondary amenorrhoea. These patients have a very brief stay in hospital, seldom having complications of any type, but should be warned that after the operation they now have a good chance of achieving normal fertility, and should use contraception if they do not wish to start a family immediately. Our clinic has two patients who became pregnant within weeks of surgery and never had a period post-operatively.

Cushing's. As mentioned above, cured patients have an absolute need for cortisol replacement following their successful surgery. They undergo significant changes during their post-operative inpatient stay, and should be warned about these changes. The earliest changes may include an improvement of vision (possibly through loss of corneal oedema) and loss of body water, which may be interpreted as partial DI. Longer-term changes include a fall in blood pressure towards normal, thinning of the face and loss of facial hair, loss of coloration of striae, flaking of the skin and restoration of normal body contours with strengthening of the thighs and thinning of the abdomen. Occasionally patients become depressed, because of the profound change in steroid status. Other patients who are significantly depressed whilst cushingoid often show a lightening of mood.

Craniotomy patients

General considerations

In general the main considerations in these patients are the same for those patients undergoing transsphenoidal surgery. Thus, all patients will be monitored for the development of DI as well as needing cortisol replacent.

Because of the risk of post-operative intracranial clots (intracerebral retraction and extradural haematomas), these patients will be nursed on the intensive care unit for 24 h, with neurological observations at 15 minute intervals for 2 hours, then half hourly for 2 hours and then hourly.

Analgesia and fluid replacement

Craniotomy is more painful than transsphenoidal surgery, and needs stronger analgesia. Most neurosurgical units in the UK will use intramuscular codeine 60 mg 3–4-hourly. Fluid replacement is as in transsphenoidal surgery and may be tailed off once the patient is drinking sufficiently. Subgaleal drains are removed at 15 minute intervals for 2 hours, then half hourly for two hours and then hourly.

Fluid balance

This is measured carefully as for transsphenoidal surgery, with the same indicants and caveats with regard to the developement of DI. In transcranial surgery the pituitary stalk is at greater risk from operative damage, and the incidence of DI is consequently very much higher—as high as 60%.[1]

Cortisol replacenent

Patients undergoing craniotomy are given dexamethasone 4 mg 6-hourly, to protect the frontal lobe and hypothalamus from the effects of retraction and dissection. This will be reduced during the first few post-operative days to a simple replacement dose of 1 mg daily. If the patient is confused, the dexamethasone reduction should be slowed down. If there are no complications, changeover to hydrocortisone 20 mg a.m. and 10 mg p.m. may be carried out on the fourth or fifth post-operative day. All patients will be discharged on replacement therapy.

CSF leaks

These are unlikely but may occur for two reasons. (1) if a transfrontal route has been used, and the frontal air sinus has been both breached and inadequately repaired, a nasal leak may occur. In this case, there is little alternative to reopening the craniotomy and closing the defect definitively, with pericranium and tissue glue. (2) The other possibility would be if there had been a previous transsphenoidal approach to the tumour and the fossa floor repair has been breached by the cranial fossa dissection. This would also present as a nasal leak, which would be repaired through a second transsphenoidal approach. Fortunately this has yet to occur to the authors' patients.

Length of stay

This is dictated by the patient's condition and the endocrine status. Once stable, the patient may safely go home. This will usually be at or about 5 or 6 days. Skin clips or sutures can be safely removed at 3 days but neurosurgical tradition usually leaves them in for 5 days.

The majority of these patients will have had optic field deficits prior to surgery and a post-operative field and acuity check is recommended, although vision if not fully recovered may continue to improve for many months following surgery.

LONG-TERM MANAGEMENT

The first follow-up is carried out at approximately 6 weeks. There are advantages if this is carried out in a multidisciplinary clinic, to allow considerations of the post-operative surgical assessment, as well as the endocrine status.

Patients who have undergone transsphenoidal surgery have few if any problems from their nose. If the mucosa was badly torn, there may be some discomfort and crusting. If a problem to the patient, it may be managed with warm saline nasal washouts. Craniotomy patients will have their operative site checked. If anticonvulsants have been used, either a decision on cessation of this therapy will be made or anticonvulsant levels will be checked.

The follow-up of the endocrine group of tumours differs considerably from those that cause mass effect problems and will be considered separately.

Endocrine tumours

Prolactinomas

The post-operative prolactin level will give a very fair idea of 'cure'.[2] If cured, at 6 weeks, many female patients of childbearing age will have shown some signs of menstruation. Hormone levels will be rechecked for thyroid function, prolactin, FSH and LH and, if male, testosterone. If the patient is still maintained on hydrocortisone, this will be referred to the attendant endocrinologist, who will usually request a Synacthen test 24 h after the withdrawal of hydrocortisone, or in some centres an insulin stress test. Further endocrine details are given in the Chapter 3. Any other hormone deficiency can at this stage be replaced. Long-term follow-up may be referred back to an endocrine clinic, especially if the prolactin has fallen to the normal range, and if the prolactin remains normal the patient can be discharged as cured.

Cure rates for surgical procedures for microprolactinomas are given in

Table 8.1 Surgical cure rates in operative series for prolactinoma

Reference	Patient numbers	Percentage cure and observations
10	50	68% micro./17% diffuse expansion/17% invasive (bromocriptine pre-treatment)
11	35	74% 0 recurrence at 5 years Hemilobectomy carried out always
12	–	80–85% 50% recurrence free at 5 years
13	100	76% if pre-op. prolactin < 22 ng/ml 39% if < 200 ng/ml
14		50% recurrence at 5 years

Table 7.1. Although good results are expected, the recurrence rate may be significant in the long term. Disturbance of the normal release of inhibiting factors through post-operative 'scarring' of the portal system may cause a partial stalk effect, with prolactin levels slightly above normal. A normal menstrual cycle can be achieved, as well as pregnancy, under these circumstances.

Recent work[3] suggests that 73.7% of patients who achieve normal prolactin levels following surgery maintain these levels for 10 years.

If the operation fails to achieve normal prolactin levels, a more difficult decision process is posed. If a normal menstrual cycle returns and the prolactin levels are only marginally raised, it is safe to pursue an expectant policy, and follow the patient at 6-month intervals. If amenorrhoea persists, hypo-oestrogenization is a significant problem which needs to be addressed Repeat surgery is a possibility, especially if a post-operative scan reveals significant residual tumour. On the other hand, bromocriptine requirements are often lower if the residual tumour fragments are not big enough to be imaged, and previous intolerance to the drug may be reversed. The role of radiotherapy will be discussed in Chapter 9.

In patients with macroprolactinomas, the main consideration will be the state of their vision. Although the prolactin level is of interest, it is not the most important factor as it is likely to remain high, and it is the cortisol and thyroid function which is of more importance in these patients. A follow-up scan will be required to assess the residual tumour volume.

Male patients who remain hypogonadal will require male hormone replacement (Sustanon given as a depot injection on a 3–4-weekly basis) unless they are elderly and find the return of sexuality troublesome. If they wish to establish fertility, the patient will need referral to a reproductive endocrinology/fertility clinic for gonadotrophin injections. If the tumour is bromocriptine sensitive, the patient can have the residual controlled by the minimum dose that will reduce this to normal; if not, radiotherapy will be necessary.

Table 8.2 Surgical cure rates in operative series for acromegaly

Reference	Patient Numbers	Cure (%)	Tumour size cure rate (%)	
			Micro.	Macro.
15	90	79	84	77
16	140	62	Not stated	
17	56	46	Not stated	
18	100	60	Not stated	
19	169	70	76	64
20	204	57	Not stated	
21	222	71	81	65

After Fahlbusch et al.[20]

Acromegaly

At 6 weeks, if the patient is cured there will be significant change in face, body and extremities. The response of GH to glucose at the time of discharge should give an indication of cure, though this or a simple profile of GH every 30 min for 2 h should be repeated, and insulin-like growth factor 1 (IGF-1) levels checked.

The likelihood of cure relates to size of tumour at the time of diagnosis. As the development of the condition is insidious, many patients have tumours that fill the fossa, or are even macroadenomas causing mass effect problems. Cure rates from various large series are given in Table 8.2.

If the tumour is incompletely removed, it is important to pursue normalization of GH secretion, as uncontrolled acromegaly leads to a high incidence of heart disease and there is some evidence for increased cancer rates. In the case of incomplete removal of tumour, the first action must be to obtain further high-quality imaging to identify residual tumour, and consider repeat surgery. Cure rates from second-time surgery are, understandably, less good than at the first time. If a tumour loculus can be identified, a second approach is worthwhile, paticularly if within a short period of the first operation. The alternative is radiotherapy, whose curative effect may take many months. Whilst awaiting a radiotherapy cure, the patient should have symptomatic control with somatostatin. At present there is little enthusiasm for long-term somatostatin therapy, although trials of depot somatostatin are under way, and represent a worthwhile alternative in some patients.

Cushing's tumours

At first follow-up, there should be a considerable change towards normal if the patient is cured. The immediate post-operative cortisol levels will have to be repeated even if the cortisol level was below 50 mg/ml, which is

Table 8.3 Surgical cure rates in operative series for Cushing's tumours

Reference	Patient Numbers	Cure rate	Comments
22	56	45/53(84.9%)	Total hypophysectomy in 9
23	28	21/26(75%)	
24	221	164/216(76%)	173 tumours, 25 total hypophysectomy
25	101	71/96(74%)	Selective adenectomy only.
25	8	4/8	Total hypophysectomy as second procedure

accepted as indicating a cure. Patients will be reassessed for their cortisol status as has been outlined in Chapter 3.

If cured, further follow-up may be at an endocrine clinc, where other aspects of pituitary function, damaged by surgery or the Cushing's disease, can be assessed. These will include fertility and thyroid function.

If there is continued activity of the tumour, a second surgical approach may be warranted if either an adenoma was found at the first procedure, particularly if a tumour residuum can be seen on a follow-up scan, or if a microadenoma supposedly found at surgery is found to be normal pituitary on histological analysis. If not, control of the disease must be obtained by bilateral adrenalectomy, followed by radiotherapy to the pituitary, to prevent the long-term development of Nelson's syndrome.

Cure rates are dependent on identification of a tumour at surgery. Reported results are given in Table 8.3.

Macroadenomas causing mass effect

Neither transsphenoidal nor transcranial surgery can effect total tumour removal of macroadenomas, except in unusual circumstances. The structures adjacent to the tumour margins prevent the type of dissection that would include the removal of a tumour-free zone and there is no true tumour capsule. Histological assessment of dura taken at surgery shows that dural invasion occurs in 94% of suprasellar tumours and 69% of microadenomas.[4] The operation is very likely to have achieved the aims of reducing the tumour bulk, and thus its mass effect on vision will have been lessened, but at some stage the chance of recurrence is high. Long-term management is directed at establishing (1) the state of vision and (2) controlling the residual effects of the tumour and the surgery on endocrine function, whilst (4) anticipating further tumour growth by either accepting the eventual need for further surgery or offering radiotherapy as a means of further reducing tumour residuum and incidence of regrowth.

Recurrence rate is very difficult to predict. In a long-term follow-up of non-functioning tumours with a mean follow-up of 73 months, Ebersold et al[5] found a 16% recurrence rate, although only six were symptomatic. With improved imaging this rate would undoubtedly be higher. The majority of tumours are indolent and cause very little short or medium-term problem; however, seemingly innocuous tumours of benign histological appearance, identical to the 'indolent' majority, can display an alarming growth rate. Tumour growth markers such as the monoclonal antibody Ki 67 may provide some answer as there is some correlation with the tumours expected to grow rapidly, such as those with aggressive Cushing's disease or Nelson's syndrome, and numbers of cells in actual replication,[6,7] but there is no simple solution to their identification at present.

Although it might be assumed that the simplest answer would be to give post-operative radiotherapy to every patient with a large tumour, successful surgical clearance or not, there are well-recognized problems associated with this strategy, which will be discussed in detail in Chapter 9. These are, in short, diminution of intellectual capacity, optic pathway radiation damage, late-onset radiation-induced pituitary failure at 10–15 years, second tumour induction[8] and failure to control regrowth. Radiotherapy is generally well-tolerated except in elderly patients, who do appear to have more problems with the treatment. Consequently, the elderly or the very young are not usually given this treatment, the latter group because of the long-term problems that will be induced during an otherwise normal age span.

Vision

Transsphenoidal surgery is very successful at restoring vision with minimal morbidity. Those patients presenting with minor field loss and acuity change should expect a return of their vision towards normal, regardless of age, size of tumour and length of history. Those with more severe loss and those with long histories, especially if associated with marked optic atrophy, may recover less of their vision. If the vision is so badly damaged that acuity and fields are minimal or absent, then prognosis of return of function must be guarded. Nevertheless, even in this group there may be significant improvement, and some may recover full vision.

Recovery rates of vision are compared in a number of series in Table 8.4. All are following transsphenoidal surgery other than the out-

Table 8.4 Recovery of vision: surgical series results

Reference	Number	Recovery and type	Comments
1	101	57% full, 37% partial	Giant and recurrent tumours excluded
26	100	79% acuity, 74% fields	Best overall data
27	34	85% improved	Complex field assessment
28	62	16.7% full, 69% improved	
29	67	Fields: 34% full, 43% partial	Acuity: 13.4% normal, 31% improved

Note: no series are directly comparable, as all use different methods of assessment. Furthermore, the make-up of each series is different.

standing transcranial series of Symon and Jacubowski, illustrating the results that can be achieved transcranially in expert hands.

Endocrine function

Anterior lobe function has a good chance of remaining unaffected if the patient enters surgery with normal function. Fahlbusch describes the normal part of the gland squashed flat over the dome of the suprasellar tumour as 'like strudel dough', so that it may be reconstituted once decompression is achieved. In our series of 67 patients presenting with visual signs from optic chiasmal compression from macroadenomas, 83.7% retained normal function, although overall the percentage is far less (61.2%) as many patients present with one or more anterior hormone deficiencies. If there is pan-hypopituitarism prior to surgery, there is no chance of restoration of any function. (Nelson[8] and author's series).

Longer-term follow-up

Once the 'immediate' treatment of the patient is complete, including surgery and radiotherapy if given, and the endocrine status returned to normal with or without replacement, the longer-term review must be considered.

Patients who presented with endocrine syndromes who have been cured may be followed up on an annual basis either by endocrinology clinics or general practitioners, using baseline hormone assays. This is necessary as there is a small annual recurrence in the 'cured' group. It is also important to remember that the patient who has had radiotherapy is likely to develop further pituitary insufficiency over the ensuing years.

Tumours causing mass effects, particularly those with hormone deficiencies, should undergo regular review. This is best carried out in a multidisciplinary clinic, where all aspects may be considered together, otherwise the patient spends a cosiderable period of time attending single clinics where the relevant details of the other clinics' decisions are inevitably missing. Once stable, review is carried out every 18 months at this institution. If the eye fields are stable there is no need for regular check, and a 2–3-yearly magnetic resonance imaging can be used to check for tumour regrowth. If there is known regrowth, then the actual decision on further surgery or radiotherapy is, in the main, predicted by the status of the eye fields alone.

REFERENCES

1. Symon L, Jakubowski J. Transcranial management of pituitary tumours with suprasellar extension. J. Neurol Neurosurg Psychiatry 1979; 42: 123–133.
2. Grossman A, Besser M. Prolactinomas. Br Med J 1985; 290: 182–184.

3. Thompson AJ, Davis DL, McLaren EH, Teasdale GM. 10 year follow up of patients with micro-prolactinoma treated by transsphenoidal surgery. Br Med J 1984; 309: 1409–10.
4. Selman WR Laws ER, Scheithauer BW, Carpenter SM. The occurrence of dural invasion in pituitary adenomas. J Neurosurg 1986; 64: 402–407.
5. Ebersold MJ, Quast LU, Laws ER. Long term results in transsphenoidal removal of non-functioning pituitary adenomas. J Neurosurg 1986; 64: 713–719.
6. Landolt AM, Subata T, Kleilus P. Growth rate of human pituitary adenomas. J Neurosurg 1987; 67: 803.
7. Nagashima T, Murovic JA, Hoshimo T et al. The proliferative potential of human pituitary tumors in situ. J Neurosurg 1986; 64: 588–593.
8. Brada M et al. Risk of second brain tumour after conservative surgery and radiotherapy for pituitary adenoma. Br Med J 1992; 304: 1343–1346.
9. Nelson AT, Tucker HStG, Becker DP. Residual anterior pituitary function following transsphenoidal resection of piuitary macroadenomas. J Neurosurg 1984; 61: 577–805.
10. Hubbard JL, Sheithauer BW, Abbond CF, Laws ER. Prolactin-secreting adenomas: the pre-operative response to bromocryptine treatment and surgical outcome. J Neurosurg 1987; 67: 816–821.
11. Hall R, Richards SH, Scanlon MF, Thomas M. Letter. Br Med J 1985; 290: 1002–1003.
12. Randall RV, Laws ER, Abbrul CF et al. Transsphenoidal microsurgical treatment of prolactin producing pituitary adenomas. Mayo Clin Proc 1983; 558: 108–121.
13. Faria MA, Tindall GT. Transsphenoidal microsurgery for prolactin secreting pituitary adenomas: results in 100 women with amenorrhea and galactorrhea syndrome. J Neurosurg 1982; 56: 33–44.
14. Serri O, Rasio E, Beauregard H et al. Recurrence of hyperprolactinaemia after selective transsphenoidal adenectomy in women with prolactinaemia. N Engl J Med 1983; 309: 280–283.
15. Hardy J, Somma M. Acromegaly: surgical treatment by transsphenoidal microsurgical removal of the pituitary adenoma. In: Tindall GT, Collins WF (eds) Clinical management of pituitary disorders. New York: Raven Press, 1979; p 209.
16. Laws E, Randall RV, Abbond CF. Surgical treatment of acromegaly: results in 140 patients. In: Givens JR (ed) Hormone secreting pituitary tumours. Chicago: Year Book, 1982; p 225.
17. Teasdale GM, Hay ID, Beatsall GH et al. Cryosurgery or microsurgery in the management of acromegaly. JAMA 1982; 247: 1289.
18. Grisoli F, Leclerq T, Jaquet P et al. Transsphenoidal surgery for acromegaly: long term results in 100 patients. Surg Neurol 1985; 23: 513–519.
19. Landolt AM, Illig R, Zapf J. Surgical treatment of acromegaly. In: Lamberts SWJ (ed) Sandostatin in the treatment of acromegaly. Berlin: Springer-Verlag, 1988; p 259.
20. Ross DA, Wilson CB. Results of transsphenoidal microsurgery for growth hormone secreting pituitary adenomas in a series of 214 patients. J Neurosurg 1988; 68: 854–867.
21. Fahlbusch R, Honegger J, Buchfelder M. Surgical management of acromegaly. Endocrinol Metab Clin North Am 1992; 21: 669–692.
22. Tindall GT, Herring CJ, Clark RV et al. Cushings disease: results of transsphenoidal microsurgery with emphasis on surgical failures. J Neurosurg 1990; 72: 363–369.
23. Arnott RD, Pestell RG, McKelvie PA et al. A critical evaluation of transsphenoidal surgery in the treatment of Cushing's disease: prediction of outcome. Acta Endocrinol (Copenh) 1990; 123: 423–430.
24. Mamplan TJ, Tyrrel JB, Wilson CB. Transsphenoidal microsurgery for Cushing's disease. Ann Intern Med 1988; 109: 487–493.
25. Fahlbusch R, Buchfelder M, Muller OA. Transsphenoidal surgery for Cushing's disease. J R Soc Med 1986; 79: 262–269.
26. Cohen AR, Cooper PR et al. (1985) Visual recovery after transphenoidal removal pituitary adenomas. Neurosurgery 17, 446–452.
27. Findlay G, McFazdean RM, and Teasdale G (1983) Recovery of vsion following treatment of pituitary tumours. Acta Neurochirurgica. 68, 175–186.
28. Laws ER Jr, Trautmann JC, Hollenhorst RW (1977) Transphenoidal decompression of the optic nerve and chiasm-visual results in sixty two patients. J. Neurosurg. 46: 717–722.
29. Powell MP, The recovery of vision following transsphenoidal surgery for pituitary adenomas. Brit Journal of Neurosurgery (in press).

Radiotherapy for pituitary tumours

*Steve M. Shalet,
Domhnall J. O'Halloran*

External radiation therapy has been used in the treatment of pituitary adenomas since the early part of the twentieth century. The major objectives are to decrease hormone secretion in the hormonally active pituitary adenomas and to inhibit tumour growth.

Most experience has been gained with external pituitary irradiation although new focal radiotherapy techniques (e.g. heavy-particle pituitary radiosurgery, gamma-knife radiosurgery, linear accelerator-based focal stereotactic radiotherapy) are being explored in a few centres.

This review concentrates on the efficacy and side-effects associated with external pituitary irradiation for pituitary adenomas, hormonally active and inactive, and craniopharyngioma, as well as discussing the therapeutic place of radiotherapy in the management of these tumours.

PROLACTINOMA

External radiotherapy is effective in reducing serum prolactin levels in patients with macroadenomas, particularly where the hyperprolactinaemia is due to true tumour hypersection, but normal levels may take over 10 years to achieve.[1] In the Manchester series of 58 hyperprolactinaemic adults with pituitary tumours there was a markedly greater response to external radiotherapy (52 patients received a dose of 35–42.5 Gy in 15 fractions over 20–22 days) in patients with positive tumour immunostaining for prolactin and/or serum prolactin concentrations above 6000 mU/l when compared with patients in whom the hyperprolactinaemia was due to stalk or hypothalamic damage.[1] A fall in serum prolactin level occurred in virtually all patients after external irradiation and life table analysis indicated a 50% probability of the serum prolactin concentration being reduced to less than 500 mU/l within 10 years.[1] The latter results compared favourably with results reported in the literature from smaller series.[2–6]

The size of the tumour is also an important prognostic factor in the effectiveness of external radiotherapy in reducing serum prolactin levels. Those patients with small tumour at presentation are more likely to achieve a prolactin level less than 500 mU/l than those with larger tumours.[1] In the series of Tsagarakis et al[7] the hyperprolactinaemic patients had predominantly small pituitary tumours and 18 out of 36 patients showed a normal serum prolactin level at a mean time of 8.5 years after radiotherapy.

One of the reasons why radiotherapy does not always bring about a normal serum prolactin level may be that external irradiation by conventional techniques also damages the hypothalamus. The hyperprolactinaemia described after external irradiation in initially normoprolactinaemic patients[8–10] is presumed to be due to hypothalamic damage and consequent impairment of dopamine neurosecretion. Interstitial irradiation with yttium-90 in similar patients does not cause hyperprolactinaemia,[11] possibly due to localization of the damage to the pituitary area.

There is little doubt that dopamine agonist therapy is the treatment of choice for patients with either large or small prolactin-secreting pituitary adenomas. However, in the uncommon hyperprolactinaemic patient with a macroadenoma who cannot tolerate dopamine agonists, radiotherapy alone or after surgery will be useful. Equally in the hyperprolactinaemic patient with a macroadenoma, in whom hypopituitarism does not reverse with dopamine agonist therapy, there will be nothing to lose by offering radiotherapy and in 50% of such patients normoprolactinaemia will be restored within 10 years. For some patients this may be a prefered alternative to lifelong dopamine agonist therapy.

ACROMEGALY

The benefits of conventional pituitary irradiation before the development of the growth hormone (GH) radioimmunoassay were judged by improved clinical and metabolic parameters. Based on these criteria it was felt that radiotherapy was more likely to be effective with a total radiation dose of greater than 35 Gy.[12] Since total doses in excess of 50 Gy were more likely to be associated with visual complications, the conventional tumour dose was set between 40 and 50 Gy. Apart from the total dose, fraction size also influences the potential risk of damage to the optic chiasm. Therefore the most commonly used regime has been a total radiation dose of 40–50 Gy in 20–25 fractions over 4–5 weeks.

Several groups have demonstrated that the GH level continues to fall for many years after radiotherapy. Thus if 'cure' is defined by the achievement of a GH level less than 10 mU/l then approximately 80% of acromegalics will be used within 10 years of irradiation.[13–15] Curiously a low-dose schedule (20 Gy in eight fractions over 11 days) produced very similar results, with 79% of patients achieving a mean GH level during glucose tolerance test (GTT) of less than 10 mU/l and 49% less than 5 mU/l within 10 years post irradiation.[16]

The initial serum prolactin level and previous surgery had no significant effect on the probability of radiation achieving a 'cure'.[16] The pre-radiotherapy GH level does, however, influence outcome in that patients with a pre-radiotherapy GH level of less than 30 mU/l show a significantly increased probability of achieving a post-radiotherapy GH level less than 5 mU/l.[16–18]

The study of the low-dose pituitary irradiation schedule was retrospective and therefore no change in radiotherapy policy is likely without 5–10-year biochemical and radiological data from a prospective randomized study comparing low-dose and conventional dose irradiation. The potential advantage of low-dose irradiation is the reduced incidence of hypo-pituitarism.[19]

The use of external radiotherapy in the treatment of acromegaly may ultimately be associated with a high incidence of clinical and biochemical resolution of the disease. Unfortunately cure following radiotherapy is slowly achieved and therefore medical therapy is valuable in ameliorating the symptoms and signs of acromegaly whilst awaiting the effects of irradiation.

The treatment of choice for acromegaly in most instances is surgery; the larger the adenoma, however, the less likely that surgery will achieve cure. Postoperatively the choice lies between radiotherapy or medical therapy with a somatostatin analogue such as octreotide. Radiotherapy is of proven benefit both in terms of tumour control and reduction in GH hypersecretion.

Octreotide appears very promising for reducing GH hypersecretion but there are no long-term data on tumour control. Therefore for most patients it is appropriate to offer radiotherapy postoperatively once lack of cure has been demonstrated biochemically. In the young acromegalic, however, still desirous of fertility and with intact gonadotrophin secretion, it may be more appropriate to offer octreotide and hold radiotherapy in reserve.

CUSHING'S DISEASE

For many years conventional external radiotherapy was the preferred treatment with prolonged remission observed in as many as 80% of patients[20] when treatment was undertaken in childhood. However, most adult series report remission rates of 40–60% with remaining patients requiring alternative therapy at a later date. Thus transsphenoidal microsurgery has now become the treatment of choice because it has the highest initial remission rate with a low incidence of complications and recurrence.

Except at very low doses, there is little relationship between the dose of irradiation delivered to the hypothalamic–pituitary axis and the overall remission rate for Cushing's disease.[21] Howlett et al[22] reported 57% drug-free remission after 45 Gy in 25 fractions over 35 days. Schteingart et al[23] found 47% in prolonged remission after 40 Gy in 20 fractions over 28 days. Ross et al[24] reported 57% remission after 46 Gy in 23 fractions over 31 days but Orth and Liddle[25] found cures in only 23% after 40–50 Gy given over a month. In a direct comparison of different dose regimes, Aristizabal et al[26] found that patients treated with total doses less than 40 Gy had a poorer response compared with those receiving higher total doses. This effect was more prominent when the daily fraction size was accounted for but their conclusions were based on small numbers, which did not achieve statistical significance. Furthermore, the results of the Manchester low-dose pituitary irradiation schedule (20 Gy in eight fractions in 11 days) with figures of 46% for initial remission and 33% for prolonged remission[27] did not support the findings of Aristizabal et al.[26]

The timing of post-treatment studies, the duration of follow-up and the criteria used to define cure will influence the remission rate, particularly in series containing late responders and late relapses. When patients in the series of Orth and Liddle[25] who responded and needed no further therapy were included, the remission rate rose from 23% to 53% but many of these patients still had abnormalities of the hypothalamic–pituitary–adrenal axis detectable by dynamic testing. Howlett et al[22] also found that only two out of 12 patients successfully irradiated (normal urinary corticosteroid levels) for Cushing's disease had normal responses to a range of dynamic test procedures as well as a normal midnight plasma cortisol level.

The best cure rate of 80% following external pituitary irradiation for Cushing's disease was achieved in children.[20] Not only is the high cure rate unmatched in any adult series but cure occurred within 18 months, which is faster than in any other series and the incidence of hypopituitarism following a conventional radiotherapy schedule was remarkably low.[20]

It was originally thought that external irradiation would prevent the development of Nelson's syndrome in previously or subsequently adrenalectomized patients with Cushing's disease. Subsequent studies were unable to support this premise and reported a similar incidence of this complication in irradiated and non-irradiated patients.[28-30] Very recently however Jenkins et al,[31] whilst confirming that pituitary irradiation does not confer absolute protection against the development of Nelson's syndrome, reported a significantly lower incidence following pituitary irradiation compared with non-irradiated. The conclusions must be tentative as the study[31] was retrospective and non-randomized. If substantiated, however, then second-line therapy for Cushing's disease in patients, who either are not cured by pituitary microsurgery or inoperable, should be external pituitary irradiation alone or in combination with bilateral adrenalectomy.

NON-FUNCTIONING ADENOMA

Recurrence of pituitary tumours after craniotomy was variably reported to be as much as 25–75%,[32–35] which led to irradiation being routinely advised after surgery performed to relieve pressure symptoms. These findings cannot, however, be extrapolated to transsphenoidal surgery.[36]

Recurrence rates after transsphenoidal surgery without irradiation for non-functioning pituitary adenomas have been reported to be between 12% and 22%.[37–39] Sassolas et al[40] reported 12% recurrence in irradiated patients and 18% in unirradiated ones within 100 months of surgery. However, these series are not homogeneous, including invasive adenomas, tumours of different size, a mixture of non-functioning and other types of adenoma and define recurrence either clinically or radiologically.

Brada et al[41] reviewed the world literature (1966–1991) on the impact of radiotherapy alone or following surgery for non-functioning pituitary adenoma. Progression-free survival ranged between 82% and 98% at 5 years, 80–95% at ten years and 72–76% at twenty years. The equivalent figures in the series of 252 patients studied by Brada et al[41] were 98%, 97% and 92% at 5, 10 and 20 years respectively. Recurrences of pituitary adenoma seen beyond 10 years suggest that a small risk of tumour progression continues regardless of the treatment approach. Brada et al[41] observed that the extent of surgical resection had no apparent influence on the long-term control; they postulate that the ultimate risk of tumour progression depends on tumour kinetics and only to a lesser extent on the amount of residual tumour. Two-thirds of their patients, however, had transfrontal surgery and as pointed out earlier it is not possible to compare the older results with transfrontal surgery with those obtained by the transsphenoidal approach. For instance, craniotomy gives poor access to the sellar contents, unlike transsphenoidal surgery which offers excellent access to the sellar contents; thus transsphenoidal surgery is more often curative.

The debate about the influence of the type of surgery on recurrence rates of non-functioning adenoma is an important one. Whilst Brada et al[41] conclude that treatment of choice should consist of limited surgical decompression followed by conventional fractionated external beam radiotherapy, Bradley et al[36] propose that a subgroup of such patients can be managed by transsphenoidal surgery alone. Bradley et al[36] studied an unirradiated group of 73 patients who showed 90% recurrence-free survival at 5 years. The subgroup identified by Bradley et al[36] were those patients who had apparently complete surgical removal as judged by the surgeon and in whom radiological or surgical evidence of spread into parapituitary structures and evidence of rapid tumour growth or histological features of invasiveness were absent. Confirmation of the surgical result with early imaging is mandatory. The major advantages of such an approach for the patient include less time off work and avoidance of further hypopituitarism and the associated reduction in quality of life.

It should, however, be pointed out that whilst the delivery of conventional external pituitary irradiation is fairly uniform throughout the UK, neuro-surgical facilities vary greatly, with only some areas possessing a 'dedicated' pituitary surgeon. Thus the operative results of transsphenoidal surgery and thus also the need for postoperative radiotherapy are likely to vary regionally. Furthermore non-functioning pituitary adenomas increase in frequency with age and are the most common of all types of pituitary adenoma in the fifth to eighth decades.[42] Therefore preservation of gonadotrophin secretion for fertility in those in whom it has not already been lost is rarely an issue.

In conclusion, patients with evidence of invasion or rapid tumour growth at the time of operation or those in whom complete removal was not carried out should be advised to have radiotherapy. In those patients who do not show such adverse features the choice lies between postoperative radio-therapy or regular clinical and radiological surveillance. A long-term pro-spective randomized trial of postoperative radiotherapy versus postoperative surveillance has not been performed. Thus patient, endocrinologist and neurosurgeon are still forced to make that decision in the absence of com-plete data.

CRANIOPHARYNGIOMA

For many years the optimum therapeutic approach to the patient with a craniopharyngioma has remained controversial. The major choices are radi-cal surgery alone or partial surgical resection followed by radiotherapy. In this context the sole purpose of the radiotherapy is to reduce the risk of clinical recurrence. In children, radical surgery carries the potential risk of inducing significant impairment of psychological and IQ status–deficits which are rarely documented in detail.

Unfortunately a prospective randomized study of these two therapeutic approaches has never been carried out. Furthermore the nature of the surgical skill involved must imply considerable variability in the surgeon's capacity to perform radical surgery, in contrast to the consistency of radio-therapy which involves fairly standard dosage schedules, radiation fields and equipment. The existing literature contains predominantly retrospective single-centre studies.

If subtotal removal is carried out, there is a 60% symptomatic recurrence rate.[43,44] In this situation the place of routine postoperative radiotherapy is now overwhelming. Bloom et al[45] treated 46 children and 66 adults with conservative surgery and radiotherapy. The 5- and 10-year survival rates for children were 85% and 74% respectively and for adults were 74% and 60% respectively. Sung et al[46] reported results in 109 patients, 74 treated by surgery alone with 5- and 10-year survival figures of 63% and 48% respectively. For 32 patients treated at the same institute by combined surgery and radiotherapy, however, the survival rates were 82% and 71% respectively, being particularly good for children.

There would appear to be a dose–response relationship which is age-dependent.[46,47] Thus in certain departments a greater total radiation dose is used for craniopharyngioma in adults compared with children. In a large series of 125 patients with craniopharyngioma, Manaka et al[48] studied 45 patients treated by surgery and postoperative radiotherapy and 80 patients who only underwent surgery. The 5- and 10-year survival results were 35% and 27% respectively (surgery alone) versus 89% and 76% (surgery and radiotherapy). The mean survival of the irradiated group was more than 10 years whereas it was 3.12 years for patients who had not received radiotherapy.

Cystic craniopharnyngioma may be treated with intracavitary brachytherapy,[49,50] which consists of instilling a radioisotope intracystically in order to deliver a large dose of irradiation to the cyst wall secretory epithelium. Yttrium-90 is a commonly chosen radioisotope and being a β-emitter the dose of irradiation reaching the optic pathways is not excessive. Some groups use an intracavitary brachytherapy procedure as primary treatment,[50] whilst others reserve this technique for a cystic recurrence in a patient who has already undergone neurosurgical resection and external irradiation.

There is often a long interval between the onset of symptoms and the diagnosis of carniopharyngioma in children, few of whom reach medical care because of symptoms of hormonal deficiency, although 83% of the children studied by Thomsett et al[51] had at least one hypothalamic–pituitary hormone deficit before treatment. GH deficiency is common; approximately half the children are short for their age and the majority show an impaired growth velocity. In addition a high proportion of these children are obese at the time of treatment and hypogonadism is also common but difficult to quantify before puberty, Adrenocorticotrophic hormone (ACTH) and thyroid-stimulating hormone (TSH) deficiencies are less common (20–30%) and a minority may show precocious puberty, while in contrast to pituitary adenomas, diabetes insipidus is relatively common owing to involvement of the supraoptic nucleus (20–30%). Additional pituitary hormone deficits occur frequently following surgery alone or combined with radiotherapy.

COMPLICATIONS OF RADIOTHERAPY

Potential adverse effects of megavoltage X-ray therapy of pituitary adenoma include hypopituitarism, visual impairment, brain necrosis and radiation oncogenesis. Hypopituitarism is numerically the most significant and the other complications are rare events.

Radiation oncogenesis

Pituitary adenomas are among the few non-malignant tumours which are regularly subjected to therapeutic irradiation; in assessing the impact of radiation on second tumour development many have followed, with modifications, the criteria laid down by Cahan et al[52] for radiation-induced bone sarcoma: evidence that the initial and second neoplastic disorders were of different cell lineage, that the second neoplastic disorder arose in the area included within the radiation beam and a long latent period of at least 3 years had elapsed before the appearance of the new tumour.

In recent years, instances of sellar fibrosarcoma, osteogenic sarcoma, meningioma and glioma have been reported after pituitary irradiation, mainly as individual case reports and rarely with any indication of the 'denominator' of incidence. The problems of statistical analysis are difficult, for the sequential tumours are rare and of a number of separate tumour species, each correspondingly rarer and with its own specific propensity for development.

An extensive review of the world literature by Jones[53] revealed 30 cases of parasellar fibrosarcoma described between 1959 and 1992. These tumours followed 2–27 years after irradiation and none was described in an un-irradiated patient. Only nine cases, however, have been reported after modern megavoltage therapy. There were 16 cases of meningioma after radiotherapy reported between 1970 and 1992 with latencies of 8–32 (median 20) years compared with 19 cases without irradiation. Similarly there were 18 cases of glioma reported post irradiation (median latency 9 years) between 1983 and 1992 compared with nine without irradiation. Radiation induction has thus been established for fibrosarcoma and to a lesser extent for meningioma and glioma but only one case of osteogenic sarcoma has been recorded after modern treatment.

There are only two clinical radiation oncogenesis studies in the literature based on substantial numbers. Jones [54] reported a series of 332 consecutive cases of pituitary adenoma, all irradiated by the uniform method of megavoltage irradiation (45 Gy per 25–26 fractions per 35 days) and reviewed after periods of 7–27 (median 18) years. No case of fibrosarcoma was encountered. There was one of glioma but also one in a parallel unirradiated patient and there was no instance of meningioma.

In the series from the Royal Marsden Hospital, however, Brada et al[55] found, among 334 patients, five cases (two glioma, two meningioma and one meningeal sarcoma) and compared this incidence with the population rates in the South Thames Region. On the basis of their own data alone, Brada et al[55] went on to suggest that there was an excess of 2.4 brain tumours per 100 patients so treated and followed for 20 years.

The occurrence of only five tumours in 666 patients reported in these two series emphasizes the rarity of these second tumours and the difficulty of interpreting small numbers especially in the absence of an appropriate control series. Furthermore it is not justifiable to amalgamate figures of the three types of radiogenic tumour in an attempt to increase total numbers of extrapolation.

The patterns of oncogenesis in even these two large series emphasize that such second tumours are rare but their true incidence could only be obtained from much larger experience.

Brain necrosis

Late necrosis of the brain, occurring between 3 months and 5 years after irradiation, has been extensively documented[56-58] and following pituitary irradiation it is most likely to affect, for reasons of dose distribution, the temporal lobes and brain stem. In clinical terms, the temporal lobe lesions are often bilateral and the presentation may be dominated by confusion and memory deficit. The lesions consist pathologically of areas of necrosis, demyelination and gliosis, with haemorrhage, vascular hyalinoid necrosis, endothelial proliferation and extravasation into the neural parenchyma.[57] The effect of both total dose and fractionation is emphasized in the report by Fujii et al[59] who found delayed brain injury in 5/25 patients receiving more than 60 Gy, 1/29 receiving 50–59 Gy and none below the 50 Gy level. This effect was compounded by four of the six affected patients having also received fractions of 3 Gy; furthermore all radiotherapy protocols consisted of co-axial fields.

The balanced three-field technique with detailed isodosimetry is designed to minimize the dose to temporal lobes and brain stem. The use of two opposed (co-axial) fields with low-megavoltage energies inevitably means that parts of the temporal lobes receive an even greater dose than the pituitary; an additional 8% for 4 MV linear accelerator radiation and 15% for radiocobalt. In cases planned to receive a target dose of 50 Gy this could amount to temporal lobe doses of 54 and 57.5 Gy respectively.[53] Previous radiotherapy techniques with only one field irradiated per day would have further increased the temporal lobe doses.

The use of modern neuroradiological techniques such as high-resolution computed tomography (CT) and magnetic resonance (MR) imaging have provided a new means of diagnosing brain necrosis.[60] These radiological findings might be associated with little or no demonstrable neurological dysfunction. Up to now, definitive evidence of radionecrosis has depended on histopathology and the significance of low-grade MR changes in this connection has yet to be established.

The possible radiotherapeutic factors in temporal lobe deficit include high radiation dose, abnormal fractionation, lack of detailed isodosimetry, irradiation by opposed fields at low megavoltage energy and use of a single field per dose.

It is important to emphasize that with modern three-field technique, detailed isodosimetry, and a maximum radiation dose of 45 Gy with due attention to fractionation, Jones[53] observed no case of brain necrosis in the series of 332 cases of pituitary adenoma irradiated between 1961 and 1982 and reviewed in 1988.

Visual impairment

The differential diagnosis of visual impairment in a patient previously irradiated for a pituitary tumour includes progressive or recurrent tumour, radiation damage to the visual pathways, particularly the chiasm, and arachnoidal adhesions around the chiasm.

Radiation-induced optic neuropathy typically presents after a latency period of 2–36 months, often with painless visual loss which progresses rapidly over days or weeks. MR imaging appears to be the most useful investigation, particularly with gadolinium enhancement.[61,62] The degree of enhancement is in keeping with a vascular aetiology. Susceptibility to radiation-induced optic neuropathy may be increased by the pressure on the optic chiasm from adjacent tumour at the time of presentation. Similarly it has been proposed that certain types of pituitary adenoma, GH- and ACTH-secreting, are more frequently associated with radiation-induced optic neuropathy, with the possible enhanced susceptibility being mediated through a hypertensive mechanism. Proof, however, is lacking.

Undoubtedly the major factors in pathogenesis are total radiation dose and fractionation schedule. The vast majority of cases of radiation-induced optic neuropathy have been described following a radiation dose in excess of 45–50 Gy.[63] Similarly very few cases have been described following a schedule which did not exceed a daily fraction of 2 Gy.[63-69]

If these guidelines are adhered to, then the risk of optic tract necrosis is very rate.[53] The occasional sporadic occurrence of this complication amongst those treated with a schedule employing these guidelines may reflect increased individual radiosensitivity.[60,61,70-72]

Radiation-induced hypopituitarism

Early studies of endocrine deficiency after radiotherapy for pituitary tumours were largely restrospective and thus the exact aetiology of any deficiency detected could not be clearly established. Pistenma et al[73] described 62 patients treated for chromophobe adenoma and found that the number requiring hormone replacement therapy increased from 30% before surgery and radiotherapy (44–70 Gy in 4.5–7 weeks) to 65% afterwards. However, this increase was attributed entirely to the surgical procedure. Subsequent small retrospective series of acromegalic patients were noted to have an increased incidence of anterior pituitary hormone deficits after radiotherapy.[74-76] Prospective studies revealed that endocrine deficiencies may develop at any time after radiotherapy for pituitary disease and that the cumulative incidence of deficiencies increases with time for at least 10 years after therapy.[13,15,17,77]

The degree of pituitary hormonal deficit is related to the radiation dose received by the hypothalamic–pituitary axis. Thus after lower radiation doses, isolated GH deficiency ensues, whilst higher doses may produce panhypopituitarism. The marked sensitivity of the hypothalamic–somatotroph axis was confirmed by the findings of Grossman et al[78] who showed an increase in the incidence of GH deficiency from 24% before radiotherapy (45 Gy per 25 fractions per 35 days) to 79% at 3 years in a group of 36 women treated for prolactinoma. In the same series Grossman et al[78] did not find a single patient who developed ACTH deficiency after therapy and only one who required thyroxine replacement.

In our own centre[10] we studied 165 adults who underwent external irradiation to the hypothalamic–pituitary region (37.5–42.5 Gy per 15–16 fractions per 20–22 days) for treatment of a pituitary adenoma (84%) or suprasellar tumour (16%). Before irradiation 79% of patients were gonadotrophin deficient; by 5 and 8 years after irradiation the incidence of gonadotrophin deficiency had risen to 91% and 96% respectively. This compares with 8-year post-irradiation incidences of 100% GH deficient (82% deficient pre irradiation), 84% ACTH deficient (41% deficient pre irrdiation) and 49% TSH deficient (20% deficient pre irradiation).

In the patients who developed multiple pituitary hormone deficiencies following irradiation the most usual order of loss of anterior pituitary hormone function was GH followed by gonadotrophins, ACTH and then TSH.[10] This sequence was seen in 61% of the patients who developed multiple pituitary hormone deficiencies, although 25% of patients with nonfunctioning pituitary adenomas and 36% of patients with acromegaly who developed multiple deficiencies developed ACTH deficiency before gonadotrophin deficiency.[10]

The development and speed of onset of pituitary hormone deficits following irradiation is dose-dependent (range 20–45 Gy). For gonadotrophins, ACTH and TSH there was a significantly greater incidence of deficiency with increasing total radiation dose.[19] Hyperprolactinaemia was seen with all the dose schedules used[19] but there was no relationship between the degree of hyperprolactinaemia and the total dose of radiation administered. In this extensive series (251 patients) we have not observed a single case of radiation-induced diabetes insipidus.[19]

Furthermore the pre-irradiation pituitary hormone status influences the timing of onset of radiation-induced pituitary hormone deficit, as illustrated by the evolution of radiation-induced GH deficiency.[79] This information may enable the clinician to predict the frequency and timing of pituitary hormone deficiency in patients irradiated for pituitary tumours and the potential need for replacement therapy.

Among patients with pituitary adenomas treated by the implantation of yttrium-90 into the pituitary gland with radiation doses of 500–1500 Gy to the pituitary, the combined incidence of TSH and ACTH deficiency was 39% at 14 years[80] as compared with an incidence of over 90% at 10 years among patients who underwent external irradiation at doses ranging from 37.5 to 42.5 Gy.[10] The most likely explanation for the difference in the incidence of hypopituitarism after the two types of irradiation is that the fields for external irradiation included the hypothalamus, which was relatively unaffected by yttrium-90 treatment.

Further evidence that the hypothalamus is the site of radiation-induced damage comes from studies in patients who have received cranial irradiation. Not only do they show (i) increased prolactin concentrations, but also (ii) those patients with gonadotrophin and TSH deficiencies show the hypothalamic damage pattern of delayed anterior pituitary hormone responses to gonadotrophin-releasing hormone (GnRH) and TRH respectively and (iii) those patients with subnormal GH response to the hypothalamic stimuli of arginine or insulin-induced hypoglycaemia and reduced spontaneous GH secretion show normal GH responses to single bolus doses of growth hormone-releasing hormone (GHRH). These are all characteristic hormonal findings in patients with pathologically documented hypothalamic disease. Furthermore there is now some evidence to suggest that direct injury of hypothelamic neurones rather than reduced cerebral blood flow is the major cause of progressive hypothalamic–pituitary dysfunction after fractionated cranial irradiation.[81]

The observation that the hypothalamus rather than the anterior pituitary gland is the site of radiation damage is of more than academic interest. It may be a physiological advantage to treat gonadotrophin deficiency with pulsatile GnRH[82] rather than exogenous gonadotrophins. Similarly there may be practical advantages to treating GH deficiency with either GHRH analogues, especially if a depot preparation becomes available, or GH-releasing hexapeptides administered orally, rather than by a daily subcutaneous injection of GH.

THE FUTURE

This review has concentrated on the impact and role of conventional radiotherapy for pituitary tumours. Recently there has been increasing interest in focal radiotherapy techniques such as proton beams, cobalt gamma-knife radiosurgery and linear accelerator focal stereotactic technology. The attractiveness of these techniques lies in their theoretical ability to deliver a high radiation dose to the tumour with much greater sparing of normal tissue. In reality the techniques are only available in a limited number of centres and the theoretical promise may not always be achieved. Almost all focal radiotherapy techniques use relatively few fractions of large size; thus if the tumour is close to the optic chiasm or other important nervous system tissues, then the latter will not be spared high-dose fraction radiotherapy. It is likely that such focal radiotherapy techniques will be reserved for carefully selected pituitary tumours.[83–85]

REFERENCES

1. Littley MD, Shalet SM, Reid H, Beardwell, CG, Sutton ML. The effect of external pituitary irradiation on elevated serum prolactin levels in patients with pituitary macroadenomas. Q J Med 1991; 81: 985–998.

2. Nabarro JDN. Pituitary prolactinomas. Clin Endocrinol 1982; 17: 129–155.
3. Mehta AE, Reyes FI, Faiman C. Primary radiotherapy of prolactinomas; 8–15 years follow-up. Am J Med 1987; 83: 49–58.
4. Johnston DG, Hall K, Kendall-Taylor P et al. The long-term effects of megavoltage radiotherapy as sole or combined therapy for large prolactinomas: studies with high definition computerised tomography. Clin Endocrinol 1986; 24: 676–685.
5. Antunes JL, Housepian EM, Frantz AG et al. Prolactin-secreting pituitary tumours. Ann Neurol 1977; 2: 148–153.
6. Gomez F, Reyes FI, Faiman C. Nonpuerperal galactorrhoea and hyperprolactinaemia. Am J Med 1977; 62: 648–659.
7. Tsagarakis S, Grossman A, Plowman PN et al. Megavoltage pituitary irradiation in the management of prolactinomas: long-term follow-up. Clin Endocrinol 1991; 34: 399–406.
8. Shalet SM, MacFarlane IA, Beardwell CG. Radiation-induced hyperprolactinaemia in a treated acromegalic. Clin Endocrinol 1979; 11: 169–171.
9. Clark AJL, Mashiter K, Goolden AW, Joplin GF. Hyperprolactinaemia after external irradiation for acromegaly. Clin Endocrinol 1982; 17: 291–295.
10. Littley MD, Shalet SM, Beardwell CG, Ahmed SR, Applegate G, Sutton ML. Hypopituitarism following external radiotherapy for pituitary tumours in adults. Q J Med 1989; 70: 145–160.
11. Clark AJL, Chahal P, Mashiter K, Joplin GF. Lack of rise in serum prolactin following yttrium 90 interstitial irradiation for acromegaly. Clin Endocrinol 1983; 19: 557–563.
12. Sheline GE, Goldberg MB, Feldman R. Pituitary irradiation for acromegaly. Radiology 1961; 76: 70–75.
13. Eastman RC, Gordon P, Roth J. Conventional supervoltage irradiation is an effective treatment for acromegaly. Clin Endocrinol 1979; 48: 931–940.
14. Sheaves R. Pituitary irradiation for acromegaly. In: Wass JAH (ed) Treating acromegaly. J Endocrinol 1994; 103–108.
15. Feek CM, McLelland J, Seth J et al. How effective is external pituitary irradiation for growth hormone secreting pituitary tumours? Clin Endocrinol 1984; 20: 401–408.
16. Littley MD, Shalet SM, Swindell R, Beardwell CG, Sutton ML. Low dose pituitary irradiation for acromegaly. Clin Endocrinol 1990; 32: 261–270.
17. Klijn JGM, Lamberts SWJ, Van Woerkom-Eijkenboom WMH et al. Long-term follow-up after external pituitary irradiation of pituitary adenomas. In: Lamberts SWJ, Tilders FJH, Van Der Veen EA, Assies J (eds) Trends in diagnosis and treatment of pituitary adenomas. Free University Press, Amsterdam, 1984; pp. 359–372.
18. Lawrence AM, Pinksy SM, Goldfine ID. Conventional radiation therapy in acromegaly: a review and reassessment. Arch Intern Med 1971; 128: 369–377.
19. Littley MD, Shalet SM, Beardwell CG, Robinson EL, Sutton ML. Radiation-induced hypopituitarism is dose-dependent. Clin Endocrinol 1989; 31: 363–373.
20. Jenings AS, Liddle GW, Orth DN. Results of treating childhood Cushing's disease with pituitary irradiation. N Engl J Med 1977; 297: 957–962.
21. Dohan FC, Raventos A, Boucot N, Rose E. Roentgen therapy in Cushing's syndrome without adrenocortical tumour. J Clin Endocrinol 1957; 17: 8–32.
22. Howlett TA, Plowman PN, Wass JAH, Rees LH, Jones AE, Besser GM. Megavoltage pituitary irradiation in the management of Cushing's disease and Nelson's syndrome: long-term follow-up. Clin Endocrinol 1989; 31: 309–323.
23. Schteingart DE, Tsao HS, Taylor CI, McKenzie A, Victoria R, Therrien BA. Sustained remission of Cushing's disease with mitotane and pituitary irradiation. Ann Intern Med 1980; 92: 613–619.
24. Ross WM, Evered DC, Hunter P, Benaim M, Cook D, Hall R. Treatment of Cushing's disease with adrenal blocking drugs and megavoltage therapy to the pituitary. Clin Radiol 1979; 30: 149–153.
25. Orth DN, Liddle GW. Results of treatment in 108 patients with Cushing's syndrome. N Engl J Med 1971; 285: 243–247.
26. Aristizabal S, Caldwell WL, Avila J, Mayer EG. Relationship of time dose factors to tumour control and complications in the treatment of Cushing's disease. Int J Radiat Oncol Biol Phys 1977; 2: 47–54.
27. Littley MD, Shalet SM, Beardwell CG, Ahmed SR, Sutton ML. Long-term follow-up of low dose external pituitary irradiation for Cushing's disease. Clin Endocrinol 1990; 33: 445–455.

28. Wild W, Nicolis GL, Gabrilove JL. Appearances of Nelson's syndrome despite pituitary irradiation prior to bilateral adrenalectomy for Cushing's syndrome. Sinai J Med 1973; 40: 68–71.

29. Moore TJ, Dluhy RG, Williams GH, Cain JP. Nelson's syndrome: frequency, prognosis and effect of prior irradiation. Ann Intern Med 1976; 85: 731–734.

30. Kuhn JM, Proeschel MF, SSSseurin DJ, Bertagna XY, Luton JP, Girard FL. Comparative assessment of ACTH and lipotropin plasma levels in the diagnosis and follow-up of patients with Cushing's syndrome: a study of 210 cases. Am J Med 1989; 86: 678–684.

31. Jenkins PJ, Trainer PJ, Plowman PN et al. The long-term outcome after adrenalectomy and prophylactic pituitary radiotherapy in adrenocorticotropin-dependent Cushing's syndrome. J Clin Endocrinol Metab 1995; 79: 165–171.

32. Grant FC. Surgical experience with tumours of the pituitary gland. JAMA 1948; 136: 668–672.

33. Emmanual IG. Symposium on pituitary tumours: (3) Historical aspects of radiotherapy, present treatment technique and results. Clin Radiol 1966; 17: 154–160.

34. Ray RS, Patterson RH. Surgical experience with chromophobe adenomas of the pituitary gland. J Neurosurg 1971; 34: 726–729.

35. Sheline G. Treatment of non-functioning adenomas of the pituitary. Am J Roentgenol 1974; 120: 553–561.

36. Bradley KM, Adams CBT, Potter CPS, Wheeler DW, Anslow PJ, Burke CW. An audit of selected patients with non-functioning pituitary adenomas treated by transsphenoidal surgery without irradiation. Clin Endocrinol 1994; 41: 655–659.

37. Ciric I, Mikhael M, Stafford T, Lawson L, Garces R. Transsphenoidal microsurgery of pituitary macroadenomas with long-term follow-up results. J Neurosurg 1983; 59: 395–401.

38. Ebershold MJ, Quasi LM, Laws JR, Sceithauer B, Randall RV. Long-term results in transsphenoidal removal of non-functioning pituitary adenomas. J Neurosurg 1986; 64: 713–719.

39. Comtois R, Beauregard H, Somma M, Serri O, Aris-Jilwan N, Hardy J. The clinical and endocrine outcome to transsphenoidal microsurgery of nonsecreting pituitary adenomas. Cancer 1991; 68: 860–866.

40. Sassolas G, Trouillas J, Treluyer C, Perrin G. Management of non-functioning pituitary adenomas. Acta Endocrinol 1993; 129 (suppl 1): 21–26.

41. Brada M, Rajan B, Traish D et al. The long-term efficacy of conservative surgery and radiotherapy in the control of pituitary adenomas. Clin Endocrinol 1993; 38: 571–578.

42. Mindermann T, Wilson CB. Age-related and gender-related occurrence of pituitary adenomas. Clin Endocrinol 1994; 41: 359–364.

43. Cabezudo JM, Vaquero J, Areitio E, Martinez R, de Sola RG, Bravo G. Craniopharyngiomas: a critical approach to treatment. J Neurosurg 1981; 55: 371–375.

44. Weiss M, Sutton L, Marcial V et al. The role of radiation therapy in the management of childhood craniopharyngioma. Int J Radiat Oncol Biol Phys 1989; 17: 1313–1321.

45. Bloom HJG. Recent concepts in the conservative treatment of intracranial tumours in children. Acta Neurochir 1979; 50: 103–116.

46. Sung DI, Chang CH, Harisiadis L, Carmel PW. Treatment results of craniopharyngiomas. Cancer 1981; 47: 847–852.

47. Onoyama Y, Abe M, Takahashi M, Yabumoto E, Sakamoto T. Radiation therapy of brain tumours in children. Radiology 1975; 115: 687–693.

48. Manaka S, Teramoto A, Takakura K. The efficacy of radiotherapy for craniopharyngioma. J Neurosurg 1985; 62: 648–656.

49. Backlund EO. Studies on craniopharyngioma. Acta Chir Scand 1972; 138: 743–747.

50. Van Den Berghe JH, Blaanw G, Breeman WA, Rahmy A, Wijingaarde R. Intracavitary brachytherapy of cystic craniopharyngioma. J Neurosurg 1992; 77: 545–550.

51. Thomsett MJ, Conte FA, Kaplan SL, Grumbach MM. Endocrine and neurologic outcome in childhood craniopharyngioma: review of effect of treatment in 42 patients. J Pediatr 1980; 97: 728–735.

52. Cahan WG, Woodward HW, Higinbotham NL, Stewart FW, Coley L. Sarcoma arising in irradiated bone. Cancer 1948; 28: 1087–1099.

53. Jones A. Complications of radiotherapy for acromegaly. In: Wass JAH (ed) Treating acromegaly, J Endocrinol 1994; 115–125.

54. Jones A. Radiation oncogenesis in relation to the treatment of pituitary tumours. Clin Endocrinol 1991; 35: 379–397.
55. Brada M, Ford D, Ashley S et al. Risk of second brain tumour after conservative surgery and radiotherapy for pituitary adenoma. Br Med J 1992; 304: 1343–1346.
56. Fukamachi A, Wakao T, Akai J. Brain stem necrosis after irradiation of pituitary adenoma. Surg Neurol 1982; 18: 343–350.
57. Gutin PH, Leibel SA, Sheline GE. Radiation injury to the nervous system. Raven Press, New York 1991.
58. Sheline GE, Wara WW, Smith V. Therapeutic irradiation and brain injury. Int J Radiat Oncol Biol Phys 1980; 6: 1215–1228.
59. Fujii T, Misumi S, Shibasaki T, Tamura M, Hyakawa K, Miyazaki M. Treatment for delayed brain injury after pituitary irradiation. No Shinkei Geka (Neurol Surg Tokyo) 1988; 16: 241–247.
60. Al-Mefty O, Kersh JE, Routh A, Smith RR. The long-term side effects of radiation therapy for benign brain tumors in adults. J Neurosurg 1990; 73: 502–512.
61. Guy J, Mancuso A, Beck R et al. Radiation-induced optic neuropathy: a magnetic resonance imaging study. J Neurosurg 1991; 74: 426–432.
62. Hudgins PA, Newman NJ, Dillon WP, Hoffman J. Radiation-induced optic neuropathy: characteristic appearances on gadolinium-enhanced MR. Am J Neuroradiol 1992; 13: 235–238.
63. Aristizabal S, Caldwell WL, Avila J. The relationship of time–dose fractionation factors to complications in the treatment of pituitary tumours by irradiation. Int J Radiat Oncol Biol Phys 1977; 2: 667–673.
64. Harris JR, Levene MB. Visual complications following irradiation for pituitary adenomas and craniopharyngiomas. Radiology 1976; 120: 167–171.
65. Atkinson AB, Allen IV, Gordon DS et al. Progressive visual failure in acromegaly following external pituitary irradiation. Clin Endocrinol 1979; 10: 469–479.
66. Hammer HM. Optic chiasmal radionecrosis. Trans Ophthalmol Soc UK 1983; 103: 208–211.
67. Bloom B, Kramer S. Conventional radiation therapy in the management of acromegaly: secretory tumours of the pituitary gland. In: Black PM et al (eds) Progress in endocrine research and therapy (Vol 1). Raven Press, New York 1984; pp 179–190.
68. Macleod AF, Clarke DG, Pambakian H, Lowy C, Sonksen P, Collins CD. Treatment of acromegaly by external irradiation. Clin Endocrinol 1989; 30: 303–314.
69. McCollough WM, Marcus RB, Rhoton AL, Ballinger WE, Million RR. Long-term follow-up of radiotherapy for pituitary adenoma: the absence of late recurrence after greater than or equal to 4500 cGy. Int J Radiat Oncol Biol Phys 1991; 21: 607–614.
70. Delattre JY, Poisson M, Pertuiset BF, Touati M, Duyckaerts C, Hauw JJ. Necrose des voies optiques, de l'hypothalamus et du tronc cerebral apres irradiation d'un adenome hypophysaire a doses conventionnelles. Rev Neurol (Paris) 1986; 142: 232–237.
71. Roden D, Bosley TT, Fowble B et al. Delayed radiation injury to the retrobulbar optic nerves and chiasm. Ophthalmology 1990; 97: 346–351.
72. Millar JL, Spry NA, Lamb DS, Dalahunt J. Blindness in patients after external beam irradiation for pituitary adenomas: two cases occurring after small daily fractional doses. Clin Radiol 1991; 3: 291–294.
73. Pistenma DA, Goffinet DR, Bagshaw MA, Hanberry JW, Eltringham JR. Treatment of chromophobe adenomas with megavoltage irradiation. Cancer 1975; 35: 1574–1582.
74. Goldfine ID, Lawrence AM. Hypopituitarism in acromegaly. Arch Intern Med 1972; 130: 720–723.
75. Lamberg BA, Kivikangas V, Vartiainen J, Raitta C, Pelkonen R. Conventional pituitary irradiation in acromegaly. Acta Endocrinol 1976; 82: 267–281.
76. Pistenma DA, Goffinet DR, Bagshaw MA, Hanberry JW, Eltringham JR. Treatment of acromegaly with megavoltage radiation therapy. Int J Radiat Oncol Biol Phys 1976; 1: 885–893.
77. Aloia JF, Archambeau JO. Hypopituitarism following pituitary irradiation for acromegaly. Hormone Res 1978; 9: 201–207.
78. Grossman A, Cohen BL, Charlesworth M et al. Treatment of prolactinomas with megavoltage radiotherapy. Br Med J 1984; 288: 1105–1109.
79. Toogood AT, Ryder DJ, Beardwell CG, Shalet SM. The evolution of radiation-induced

growth hormone deficiency in adults is determined by the baseline growth hormone status. Clin Endocrinol 1991; 43: 97–103.
80. Jadresic A, Jimenez LE, Joplin GF. Long-term effect of ^{90}Y pituitary implantation in acromegaly. Acta Endocrinol 1987; 115: 301–306.
81. Chieng PU, Huang TS, Chang CC, Chong PN, Tien RD, Su CT. Reduced hypothalamic blood flow after radiation treatment of nasopharyngeal cancer: SPECT studies in 34 patients. Am J Nucl Radiol 1991; 12: 661–665.
82. Park KH, Park W, Lee BS et al. Pulsatile gonadotrophin-releasing hormone therapy in patients with pituitary tumours treated by surgery and irradiation. Clin Endocrinol 1994; 40: 407–411.
83. Plowman PN. Focal brain radiotherapy. J Neurol Neurosurg Psychiatry 1990; 53: 541.
84. Thomson ES, Gill SS, Doughty D. Stereotactic multiple are radiotherapy. Brit J Radiol 1990; 63: 745–751.
85. Levy RP, Fabrikant JI, Lyman JT et al. Clinical results of stereotactic heavy charged particle radiosurgery of the pituitary gland. In: Steiner L (ed) Radiotherapy: baseline and trends. Raven Press, New York 1992; pp 149–154.

10 | Parasellar lesions other than pituitary adenomas

Kamal Thapar, Ed. Laws Jr.

INTRODUCTION

Pituitary adenomas, although numerically the most significant of the sellar/ parasellar lesions, represent only one of a multitude of pathological processes occurring in the area. Converging on the modest confines of the sella turcica is an impressive number of intricate anatomical structures of neural, endocrine, vascular, osseous and meningeal origins. It is remarkable that such morphological and functional diversity can be so intimately represented in such a discrete area of the neuroaxis, and that accompanying each anatomical component is a correspondingly diverse set of pathological processes. A sprinkling of embryonic 'rests' sequestrated in the vicinity provides the substrate for various sequelae of disordered embryogenesis. Surrounding tissues of neural, meningeal and mesenchymal origins further contribute an assortment of tumour types, such that relatively few forms of intracranial neoplasia escape representation in the sellar and parasellar regions.

The myriad of pathological possibilities is further supplemented by a collection of non-neoplastic 'tumour-like' afflictions which can involve any of a variety of sellar region structures. Many of these are inflammatory in nature, ranging from acute suppuration, through chronic granulomatous conditions, to autoimmune processes. Others are structural abnormalities such as the empty sella syndrome and aneurysms of the internal carotid artery. So although pituitary adenomas may be the most common mass lesions encountered in the sellar region, a number of other pathological processes do periodically involve the area. Many of these conditions may masquerade clinically and radiologically as pituitary adenomas; both the clinician and the pathologist must always be prepared for unusual pathology when approaching lesions of the sellar and parasellar region.

In this chapter, we review the diagnosis and management of sellar and parasellar lesions, exclusive of pituitary adenomas. It is important to recognize that despite the aetiological, pathological and biological diversity of the various tumour and tumour-like conditions represented in the sellar region, most are unified by a fairly generic pattern of clinical presentation—one dominated by the predictable ophthalmological, endocrinological and neurological sequelae of a sellar region mass. Furthermore, because many of these lesions share overlapping radiological features—ones which all too frequently mimic seemingly typical pituitary adenomas—definitive pre-operative diagnoses are frequently difficult to establish with certainty. Nonetheless, such distinctions must be made, for accompanying each of the different pathological processes of the sellar region (Table 10.1) is an equally different set of diagnostic and therapeutic imperatives.

DIAGNOSIS OF SELLAR AND PARASELLAR LESIONS: GENERAL PRINCIPLES

The clinical features of sellar region pathology primarily represent the functional consequences of mass lesions which, independent of histology, compress, distort or otherwise compromise any of a variety of parasellar structures. The optic apparatus, cranial nerves of the cavernous sinus, pituitary gland, hypothalamus, ventricular system and the brain proper are all vulnerable. Given this spectrum of potential involvement, lesions arising in and around the sella require a comprehensive diagnostic approach—one in which neurological neuro-ophthalmological, endocrinological and neuro-radiological evaluations are all essential components. Each of these is fully

Table 10.1 Differential diagnosis of neoplasmas and "tumour-like" lesions of the sellar region

Tumours of adenohypophyseal origin
    Pituitary adenoma
    Pituitary carcinoma
Tumours of neuohypophyseal origin
    Granular cell tumour
    Astrocytoma of posterior lobe and/or stalk (rare)
Tumours on non-pituitary origin
    Craniopharyngioma
    Germ cell tumours
    Glioma (hypothalamic, optic nerve/chiasm, infundibulum)
    Meningioma
    Hemangiopericytoma
    Chordoma
    Hemangioblastoma
    Lipoma
    Giant cell tumour of bone
    Chondroma
    Fibrous dysplasia
    Sarcoma (chrondrosarcoma, osteosarcoma, fibrosarcoma)
    Postirradiation sarcomas
    Paraganglioma
    Schwannoma
    Glomangioma
    Esthesioneuroblastoma
    Primary Lymphoma
    Melanoma
Cysts, Hamartomas and Malformations
    Rathke's cleft cyst
    Arachnoid cyst
    Epidermoid cyst
    Dermoid cyst
    Gangliocytoma
    Empty sella syndrome
Metastatic tumours
    Carcinoma
    Plasmacytoma
    Lymphoma
    Leukaemia
Inflammatory conditions
    Infection/abscess
    Mucocele
    Lyphocytic hypophysitis
    Sarcoidosis
    Langerhans' cell histiocytosis
    Giant cell granuloma
Vascular Lesions
    Internal carotid artery aneurysms
    Cavernous angioma

discussed in the context of individual lesions throughout this and previous chapters. Issues pertaining to the endocrinology of sellar/parasellar lesions require special consideration, and they are elaborated here. Moderate degrees of hyperprolactinaemia (<6000 mU/l) can occur with any of a variety of mass lesions involving the sellar region. This phenomenon, frequently referred to as the 'stalk effect' (see Ch. 3, Medical Management), is the result of compressive or destructive lesions involving the hypothalamus or pituitary stalk. A fairly common occurrence, hyperprolactinaemia of this degree may be the result of any structural, inflammatory, or neoplastic process occurring in the sella. It is, therefore, a nonspecific finding whose presence should not be routinely interpreted as being the result of a prolactin secreting pituitary adenoma. Posterior pituitary failure in the form of diabetes insipidus is an occasional feature of sellar region pathology. Although diabetes insipidus is known to accompany a wide variety of sellar lesions, it is especially prominent in destructive processes such as granulomatous inflammation or metastic deposits to the region. Unexplained, but of practical interest, is the fact that diabetes insipidus is rarely, if ever, a presenting feature of pituitary adenomas, and its pre-operative presence strongly suggests an alternative diagnosis. The clinical features of diabetes insipidus are well known, consisting of polyuria resulting in polydipsia, and an inappropriately dilute urine in the presence of a normal or hyperosmolar plasma.

In all patients suspected of having sellar region pathology, a thorough laboratory evaluation of endocrine status is mandatory.

PRIMARY TUMOURS OF THE SELLAR REGION

Craniopharyngiomas

Representing only 3% of all intracranial tumours overall, the craniopharyngioma is nonetheless one of the more common destructive lesions of the sellar region. Virtually every aspect of craniopharyngioma biology is the subject of ongoing debate. Nagging uncertainties regarding its cellular origins, opposing surgical philosophies concerning the need for a radical approach to resection and the relative controversy over its natural history, all provide immediate stimulus for intellectual discussion.

Craniopharyngiomas are generally believed to be developmental lesions, thought to arise from remnants of Rathke's pouch. Such embryonic remnants assume the form of epithelial 'rests', deposited between the tuber cinereum and the pituitary gland, along the tract of an incompletely involuted hypophyseal–pharyngeal duct. Correspondingly, craniopharyngiomas can arise anywhere along this path.[1-3] Craniopharyngiomas could also arise from the squamous metaplasia of normal cells situated on the pituitary stalk, as was once an alternative explanation of their origin. However, evidence in favour of such a view has been conflicting.[3]

From the standpoints of size, location, contents, pathological appearance and overall clinical behaviour, craniopharyngiomas encompass a broad biological spectrum. At the one extreme are minute tumours of microscopic proportions situated wholly within a normal pituitary gland. At the other and more common extreme are larger tumours whose progressive growth enables them to compress the pituitary gland and stalk, optic apparatus and hypothalamic structures. Not infrequently, these larger lesions also extend into the third ventricle causing hydrocephalus, or permeate cerebrospinal fluid (CSF) spaces to gain access to the middle and posterior cranial fossae.

Craniopharyngiomas can be solid or cystic, and the overwhelming majority exhibit both features. The cyst contents, though classically described as 'engine oil' in appearance and consistency, can range from a shimmering cholesterol-laden fluid to a brown-black purulent sludge mixed with desquamated debris. Calcification is a common feature of cranio-pharyngiomas, ranging from microscopic specks to palpable, and even bone-like concretions. Pathologically, the epithelial elements comprising these tumours can range from cuboidal to columnar, or squamous in appearance. There has been an increasing tendency to distinguish cranio-pharyngiomas as being either classically adamantinomatous or papillary in nature.[3] Although the latter has been proposed as a distinct clinico-pathological entity, featuring a predilection for adults, a less aggressive biology and an overall favourable prognosis, so rigid a distinction may not be entirely justifiable, for papillary variants may simply reflect one component of the biological heterogeneity so characteristic of cranio-pharyngiomas in general.

Topologically, approximately 80% of craniopharyngiomas arise in and maintain a suprasellar location. These lesions are often tenaciously adher-rent to, and occasionally invasive of, the optic apparatus, hypothalamus, pituitary stalk, cranial nerves, vascular structures and surrounding brain parenchyma. Emphasis has also been placed upon the intensely gliotic nature of the brain parenchyma at the tumour–brain interface, and its suitability as a safe surgical plane facilitating tumour removal. Approxi-mately 20–30% of craniopharyngiomas originate within the sellae, resulting in its enlargement in a fashion similar to that seen with pituitary adenomas.[4] Rare examples of craniopharyngiomas wholly situated within the third ven-tricle, optic chiasm or sphenoid bone have been reported.[3]

The clinical presentation of craniopharyngiomas is determined by the age of the patient and the size and location of the tumour. In general, symptoms can be categorized as endocrine, visual, cognitive, and those deriving from increased intracerebral pressure (ICP).

Endocrine dysfunction is more conspicuous in the paediatric population and is manifested primarily by retardation of growth and sexual devel-opment. In adults, endocrine symptoms are often subtle, particularly those related to partial hypopituitarism. The effects of combined hypo-gonadotrophinaemia together with moderate hyperprolactinaemia from stalk or hypothalamic compression are generally more obvious, especially in young women, manifesting as amenorrhoea and occasionally galactorrhoea. Diabetes insipidus may coexist in all age groups.

Visual dysfunction referable to chiasmatic or optic nerve compression occurs in patients of all ages, though children are more tolerant of, and more

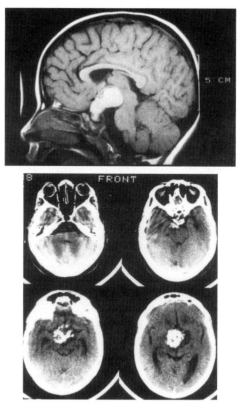

Fig. 10.1 Craniopharyngioma. Sagittal T1-weighted MRI.

difficult to test for, visual field deficits. Cognitive symptoms in the form of memory loss, dementia and psychiatric symptoms occur less frequently and are seen primarily in adults. Elevations in ICP, usually as the result of obstructive hydrocephalus, are not uncommon. Accordingly, headache, vomiting, papilloedema, ataxia and, rarely, cranial nerve palsies may all be additional presenting features.

All patients should have a comprehensive endocrine evaluation. Visual performance should be documented with fundoscopic examination, tangent screen and perimetry. With computed tomography (CT) or magnetic resonance imaging (MRI), craniopharyngiomas typically appear as inhomogeneous lesions—ones in which cystic components can often be discerned from solid elements. Calcification is often present and can be a helpful diagnostic clue (Fig. 10.1).

In newly diagnosed patients, maximum safe tumour resection is often a reasonable initial goal. In many instances, this can be achieved via craniotomy, although in selected cases transsphenoidal resection provides safer access. In others, complete excision will require a combination of both approaches. Tumours unassociated with sellar enlargement generally arise and remain suprasellar, and therefore are best managed by a transcranial (pterional or subfrontal) route. During the course of tumour resection it will usually become evident whether or not complete removal is a safe and feasible strategy. Aggressive attempts to remove tumour fragments which are tenaciously adherent to neural and vascular structures will be accompanied by an unacceptable functional cost. Alternatively, other tumours will be less adherent and complete excision can be safely achieved.

As a rule, craniopharyngiomas associated with sellar enlargement can be regarded as subdiaphragmatic in origin.[2] Even though such tumours may exhibit significant intracranial extension, they invariably maintain an 'extrapial' and 'extra-arachnoid' disposition. Accordingly, they remain amenable to complete excision via a transsphenoidal route.

The management of the recurrent craniopharyngioma is considerably more complex, for therapeutic goals must be especially well defined.[1,2,4] In some cases, and despite the technical demands of reoperation, total resection can still be achieved. However, for many recurrent tumours palliative surgery is often the most realistic goal. Recurrent lesions with a significant cystic component can often be treated by repeat aspiration. This can be achieved by inserting a silastic tube attached to an Ommaya reservoir into the cyst cavity. Alternatively, the transsphenoidal insertion of a silastic tube from the tumour cavity into the posterior nasal space can provide prolonged drainage. In addition to conventional irradiation, there are several other radiotherapeutic options applicable to recurrent tumours.[5] For cystic lesions, intracavitary instillation of radioactive solutions containing colloidal phosphorus, yttrium or gold has been of benefit. Solid recurrences have been treated with intersitial brachytherapy (the irradiation of lesions by insertion of an isotope within the tumour) and stereotactic radiosurgery.

The prognosis of craniopharyngiomas depends, in large measure, on the completeness of tumour resection. For completely excised lesions, no adjuvant therapy is required. The outlook for these patients is favourable, although late recurrence has been reported in as many as 25% of patients despite 'total' removal.[5] For incompletely resected tumours, symptomatic recurrence is virtually guaranteed, thus radiation therapy is indicated to forestall recurrence. In one recent series, 'radical subtotal resection' followed by radiotherapy provided progression-free survival in 91% of patients during a mean follow-up period of 4 years.[6] In all patients, periodic endocrine evaluation and appropriate replacement therapy are important.

Germ cell tumours

Although uncommon, germ cell tumours remain one of the principal diagnostic considerations in the evaluation of a sellar region mass, particularly in the paediatric population. In North American and United Kingdom series, germ cell tumours account for only 1% of all intracranial tumours;

however, approximately 35% of these will involve the suprasellar regions. Why these tumours should be far more common in Japan, where they account for 10% of all intracranial tumours, remains an epidemiological curiosity. Germ cell tumours typically occur during childhood and adolescence, having their peak incidence within the first two decades of life. Whereas those arising in the pineal region have a predilection for males, germ cell tumours of suprasellar origin appear notably more common in females.

It is important to recognize that germ cell tumours represent a collection of embryologically interrelated entities, each differing in germinal composition, degree of differentiation and overall biological malignancy.[7] At the most benign extreme is the mature teratoma—a well-differentiated lesion composed of mature tissues derived from all three germ cell layers. The remaining germ cell tumours are fully malignant lesions, exhibiting both local invasiveness and metastatic capability. In order of increasing biologically aggressiveness germ cell tumours include germinoma, immature teratoma, embryonal carcinoma, endodermal sinus tumour and choriocarcinoma.[7] From practical and prognostic standpoints, malignant germ cell tumours are distinguished as being either germinomas or non-germinomatous germ cell tumours. The former account for 60% of all germ cell tumours and generally have a more favourable prognosis. By contrast, non-germinomatous germ cell tumours, being neoplastic counterparts of the most primitive of primordial tissues, can be considered among the most extreme examples of human malignancy—ones which usually prove fatal despite multimodality therapy. Mixed germ cell tumours composed of both germinomatous and non-germinomatous elements have also been increasingly recognized.

Germ cell tumours involving the sellar region are usually situated in the suprasellar cistern, tenaciously adherent to, if not frankly invasive of, the basal brain surface, hypothalamus, optic nerves and pituitary stalk. Larger lesions may extend upward into the anterior third ventricle and, less frequently, downward into the sellae. Germ cell tumours of primary intrasellar origin are rare, although they have been known to cause sellar expansion, chiasmal compression and cavernous sinus invasion in a fashion similar to pituitary adenomas.[8] Synchronous lesions occurring in both suprasellar and pineal locations are present in fewer than 10% of cases.[7]

The well-known clinical triad of diabetes insipidus, visual disturbance and panhypopituitarism frequently characterizes the presentation of suprasellar germ cell tumours. Diabetes insipidus is an important diagnostic feature—one which may occasionally antedate other clinical or radiological evidence of the tumour by years. Panhypopituitarism is generally the result of hypothalamic or stalk compression, and is usually manifested as delay or regression of sexual development or growth failure. Occasionally, a prepubertal child may present with precocious puberty, a phenomenon related to either hypothalamic compression/damage or the liberation of β-human chorionic gonadotrophin (β-hCG) by the tumour. Hydrocephalus, the result of third ventricular obstruction, is generally a late finding. MRI is the radiological investigation of choice; however, germ cell tumours lack any specific radiological features which unequivocally distinguish them from other lesions (craniopharyngioma, chiasmatic glioma, hypothalamic hamartoma/glioma) occurring in the region.

Acknowledging the limitations of radiological imaging in reliably predicting tumour histology, there has been increasing use of various tumour markers as more accurate predictors of tumour histology.[9,10] α-fetoprotein (AFP), β-hCG and placental alkaline phosphatase (PLAP) as measured in both the blood and CSF are most commonly measured. Elevations of AFP suggest an endodermal sinus tumour, or a mixed tumour containing endodermal sinus elements. Elevations of β-hCG suggest a choriocarcinoma or a mixed tumour containing choriocarcinoma elements. When neither AFP nor β-hCG are elevated, a diagnosis of pure germinoma or teratoma is suspected. However, germinomas may also show variable elevations of β-hCG. Very high levels of PLAP suggest a diagnosis of germinoma; however, lesser elevations are compatible with any of the various germ cell entities. Despite their theoretical use, these tumour markers lack sufficient sensitivity and specificity to be routinely informative, and although they are frequently suggestive of tumour histology, only occasionally are they diagnostic. When elevated, however, these tumour markers are helpful in the ongoing follow-up of patients.

Although there is ongoing controversy over the optimal management of intracranial germ cell tumours in general, opinion appears less divided when suprasellar germ cell tumours are concerned.[10] The inability of MRI or tumour markers to distinguish reliably the radiosensitive germinomas from the aggressive non-germinomatous germ cell tumours or, for that matter, other more common lesions occurring in the region such as craniopharyngiomas, has placed increasing importance on obtaining a precise tissue diagnosis before instituting therapy. Accordingly, and after correction of any endocrine deficits, surgery plays both a diagnostic and therapeutic role. Except for the rare germ cell tumours of intrasellar origin which have been successfully approached transsphenoidally, most suprasellar germ cell tumours require craniotomy, usually through a subfrontal or subfrontal–pterional approach. Generous tissue sampling is obtained, the optic apparatus is decompressed, and a non-radical debulking procedure is undertaken. Except in the benign, mature teratoma when attempts at gross total excision may effect cure, there is little evidence that radical resection of malignant germ cell tumours supports any survival advantage.

Post-operatively, all malignant germ cell tumours require some form of adjuvant therapy, the nature of which is based on the histological diagnosis and the degree of disseminated disease. The frequency of metastatic dissemination among these tumours has been variably reported as being between 10% and 57%.[7] The majority of metastatic deposits occur within the neuroaxis; only 3% of all metastases occur systemically. The most important objective of staging is to exclude clinically occult subarachnoid deposits, the presence of which can be determined by studies of CSF cytology and spinal MRI. Germinomas, given their exquisite radiosensitivity, are treated with 500 rads to the tumour field, with additional craniospinal boosts should multifocal disease or positive CSF cytology be demonstrated. The prognosis of suprasellar germinomas is favourable, as contemporary series show that patient survival approaches 90% at 5 years and longer.[11,12] On the other hand, non-germinomatous germ cell tumours continue to fare far worse despite surgery and radiation therapy; only exceptional cases are alive at 5 years as most patients succumb to local recurrence within 18 months of diagnosis.[10] The effectiveness of chemotherapy for non-germinomatous germ cell tumours of the gonads has rejuvenated interest in applying the same to their intracranial counterparts. One preliminary report demonstrated that post-operative neoadjuvant chemotherapy (cisplatin and VP-16) followed by craniospinal radiation, and followed again with chemotherapy (vinblastine, bleomycin, carboplatin and VP-16) resulted in an encouraging tumour response in small series of patients.[10,13] The evolution of aggressive chemotherapeutic regimens such as this one hold much promise in the management of non-germinomatous germ cell tumours—lesions which otherwise portend a uniformly terrible prognosis.

Meningiomas of the sellar region

Approximately 10% of all intracranial meningiomas involve parasellar structures, and approximately 10% of all parasellar tumours are meningiomas. The majority are situated in the suprasellar region, taking their dural origin from the tuberculum sellae, planum sphenoidale, olfactory groove, diaphragma sellae, medial sphenoid wing, optic nerve sheath and the anterior fossa floor/orbital roof. Although intrasellar extension may be an occasional, and typically late feature of meningiomas arising at any of these sites, purely intrasellar meningiomas are exceptionally rare.[14] The majority of meningiomas involving the sellar region tend to be large circumscribed lesions which are compressive of adjacent structures. Less often, and notably in the case of sphenoid wing meningiomas, they grow in an en plaque configuration, so insinuating themselves around cranial nerves and blood vessels that surgical removal becomes a formidable challenge. Erosion, hyperostosis, or frank invasion of bone may be features of any meningioma of the skull base, although they are especially prominent in the en plaque variety. All histopathological variants of meningioma, including the aggressive angioblastic and hemangiopericytoma subtypes, are known to occur in and around the sella. Meningiomas in the parasellar region have also occurred following radiation therapy for a pituitary adenoma.

Although meningiomas situated at different parasellar sites will have, to some degree, certain unique site-specific presentation patterns,[15] some

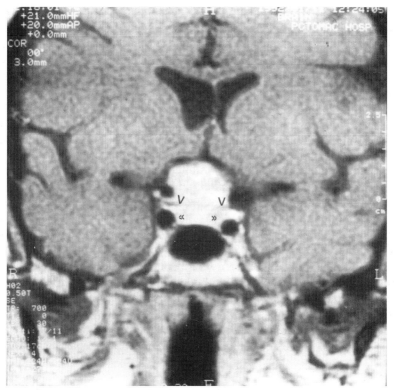

Fig. 10.2 Coronal T1-weighted MRI of a suprasellar meningioma, showing an intact diagphram separating tumour (black arrowheads) from normal gland (double arrowheads).

clinical features are common to all meningiomas occurring in the region. Insidiously progressive visual loss is a common presenting symptom (see Ch. 4, Visual Manifestations). Alterations in mental status may accompany those lesions compressing the basal frontal lobes, or those large enough to cause elevated ICP. Hypopituitarism is uncommon and generally late in occurrence. Hyperprolactinaemia on the basis of hypothalamic or pituitary stalk compression may occur, and has in some instances been associated with the amenorrhoea–galactorrhoea syndrome. Lesions involving the cavernous sinus may present varying components of a cavernous sinus syndrome.

The CT, MRI and angiographic characteristics of meningiomas are sufficiently well known that their pre-operative diagnosis can usually be made with some degree of certainty (Fig. 10.2). Of concern, however, are those rare meningiomas of intrasellar origin and occasional suprasellar meningiomas which descend into the sella causing considerable diagnostic difficulties. In such circumstances, meningiomas may be mistaken for pituitary adenomas or other intrasellar pathologies.

The operative management of meningiomas is well described elsewhere and will not be reviewed here.[15] One technical issue, however, merits emphasis and concerns those meningiomas having an intrasellar component. Such lesions, whether primarily arising within the sella or secondarily extending into it from the cavernous sinus or a more superior site, generally require a transcranial procedure for their removal. In instances where such meningiomas have been mistaken for pituitary adenomas, the transsphenoidal approach has proven somewhat of a disappointing endeavour. The inability to secure their vascular supply together with their fibrous nature which prevents their descent into the operative field complicates effective transsphenoidal removal. In such circumstances, after obtaining a frozen section diagnosis of meningioma, it is often advisable to abandon the procedure and plan a transcranial approach at a later date.

Chordomas

Chordomas are uncommon tumours of bone, presumed to arise as neoplastic derivatives of embryonal notochord remants.[16–18] Accordingly, they can arise at any site along the axial skeleton, with 35% of all cases involving the clivus. Men are usually affected twice as often as women, and curiously, despite their presumed embryonal origins, chordomas rarely affect individuals less than 20 years of age. Although chordomas appear histologically benign, this aspect of their biology has been overemphasized, for their locally destructive nature, unrelentingly progressive course and variable metastatic potential, collectively legitimize their inclusion as truly malignant tumours.

As a rule, cranial chordomas are midline lesions, and virtually all are, in some way, related to the clivus. Their precise site of origin determines their clinical presentation. Some will arise in the mid and lower clival regions producing multiple cranial nerve palsies and brain stem compression, whereas others will originate from the ventral aspect of the clivus, producing symptoms of a nasopharyngeal mass. This discussion, however, concerns those chordomas whose origin in the most rostral extreme of the clivus and dorsum sellae warrants their inclusion as a sellar region mass (basis–sphenoidale chordomas). Such lesions may extend into the sella, producing hypopituitarism or, with suprasellar extension, a chiasmal syndrome. Lateral penetration into the cavernous sinus may compromise cranial nerves transiting therein. Headache, usually the result of bony destruction, is a common accompaniment. All chordomas are locally invasive extra-axial lesions which begin with expansile bony destruction at their site of origin, followed later by infiltration and transgression of the dura, with eventual and widespread intracranial extension and encasement of cranial nerves, brain stem and vascular structures. Metastatic dissemination is usually a late occurrence— one encountered clinically in 10–20% of cases, and at autopsy in up to 40% of cases.

The radiographic appearance of chordoma, as determined by CT and

(a)

(b)

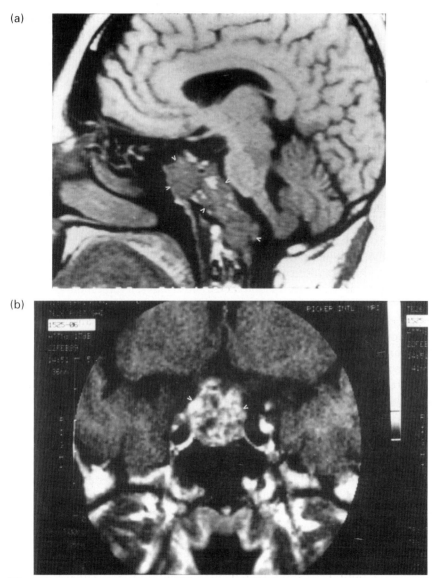

Fig. 10.3 (**a**) Sagittal and (**b**) coronal T1-weighted MRI of a rostrally extending chordoma of the clivus. Note the extensive bony destruction of the clivus (a) and the impressive seprasellar extension (b).

MRI, is fairly characteristic, consisting of a destructive and expansile process of the skull base in association with a coarsely calcified soft tissue mass (Fig. 10.3).

The combination of surgery and radiation therapy constitutes standard therapy for chordomas. However, both have significant limitation, as evidenced by the fact that the majority of patients so treated eventually succumb to recurrent local disease. Surgical access to chordomas can be provided by a variety of standard intradural and extradural approaches. Selection of the most suitable approach for any given lesion will depend primarily upon whether the tumour is midline or lateral, and whether it is intra- or extradural. For intradural, rostrally placed lesions of the parasellar region, particularly those having significant lateral, suprasellar or cavernous sinus extension, a pterional or subfrontal craniotomy provides good access to the intracranial component of the tumour. When such tumours have a significant extradural component or for basis-sphenoidal chordomas which are wholly extradural and midline, an anterior extradural approach is generally required. Accordingly, extradural involvement of the sphenoid sinus, sella or upper clivus can best be approached by the transsphenoidal route. When the areas or disease are below the anterior fossa floor, the transbasal approach of Derome provides ideal exposure.[17] Given the anatomical limits of all standard approaches, certain chordomas, depending on their particular geometry, will require combined or multiple procedures. Although gross 'total' removal is the surgical objective in most cases, it is difficult to achieve, even with the benefit of elaborate skull base operation strategies currently employed.

Radiation therapy appears to offer some measure of temporary tumour control, but because tumoricidal doses generally exceed levels of CNS tolerance, tumour recurrence has proven to be inevitable. Stereotactic techniques of radiation delivery such as a brachytherapy and radiosurgery are currently being evaluated.

As determined by various series, the mean survival of patients with chordoma ranged from 4.2 to 5.2 years.[18] The average time to first recurrence is approximately 3 years. A variant of chordoma, containing conspicuous foci of cartilaginous material interwined between tumour cells, is known as the chondroid chordoma. The variant accounts for approximately one-third of all cranial chordomas. Although its clinical presentation is indistinguishable from the standard chordoma, its prognosis is much more favourable. The mean survival of patients with chondroid chordoma is almost 16 years.

Parasellar gliomas

Mass lesions involving parasellar structures will occasionally arise from glial tissues. This is especially true in the paediatric population wherein the possibility of a glial tumour is commonly considered in the differential diagnosis of a suprasellar mass. The majority of these are astrocytomas whose anatomical origin include the optic nerve/chiasm, hypothalamus and third ventricular walls. In many instances, however, assignment of a precise anatomical origin is difficult, if not impossible, given the infiltrative nature of most astrocytic tumours and the sleek anatomical continuity of the third ventricular floor, hypothalamus and optic chiasm. Rarely, astrocytomas may arise from the infundibular stalk, and even more rarely from the posterior pituitary. Finally, occasional glial tumours such as ependymomas or choroid plexus papillomas will arise within the anterior third ventricle, secondarily descending into the surpasellar space.

Collectively, visual pathway and hypothalamic gliomas account for approximately 5% of all paediatric intracranial tumours, with most occurring during the first decade of life. Most of these lesions are low-grade astrocytomas of pilocytic type; low-grade fibrillary variants also occur, but less frequently. Rarely, and notably in the adult patient, gliomas located here tend to be higher-grade lesions—ones assuming the histology and behaviour of glioblastoma multiforme. Between 15% and 35% of patients with visual pathway gliomas will also have neurofibromatosis (NF-1).[19] Whether tumours occurring in the presence of NF-1 behave differently from sporadic ones remains uncertain.

The clinical presentation of these lesions depends primarily on their location. Diagnostic features of intraorbital tumours and intracranial tumours confined to the optic nerve include decreased visual acuity, optic atrophy, proptosis and, in the young child, strabismus and/or nystagmus. Chiasmatic–hypothalamic lesions also present with visual loss, often with bilateral field deficits. In addition, these lesions may also be accompanied by hydrocephalus and elevated ICP as the result of ventricular obstruction.

Endocrine dysfunction is frequently reported with these lesions, assuming the form of growth failure, precocious puberty and occasionally the diencephalic syndrome. Generally occurring in infants, the latter is fairly specific to processes involving the anterior hypothalamus and is characterized by failure to thrive, emaciation, hyperkinesis, nystagmus and inappropriate euphoria. The anatomical diagnosis is best provided by MRI (Fig. 10.4). The presence of a suprasellar lesion with contiguous optic nerve and/or optic tract thickening is said to be pathognomonic of an optic pathway glioma.[20]

The optimal management of these lesions remains a subject of ongoing debate. The necessity of tissue diagnosis, the indications for treatment, as well as the timing and form of intervention, are all issues steeped in controversy. Much of the uncertainty stems from the seemingly erratic natural history of these tumours. In many instances, their natural history is one of quiescence and negligible growth over long periods of time.[19] In a significant yet uncertain proportion of cases, however, their behaviour is unpredictable wherein periods of quiescence abruptly give way to progressive growth, visual and neurological compromise, and eventually patient demise.[20–23] In non-progressive lesions—ones in which the radiological diagnosis of glioma is near certain and the patient remains neurologically stable—careful observation is often prescribed as the wisest course. In progressive lesions, such as those associated with increasing neuroendocrine deficits and elevations in ICP, some form of intervention will be required. Therapeutic options include surgery, irradiation or chemotherapy. The main indication for sur-

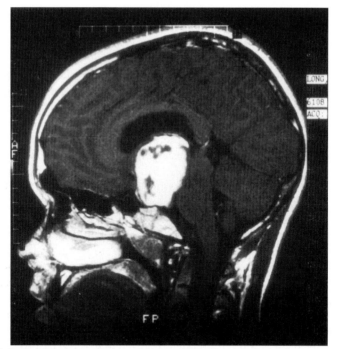

Fig. 10.4 Sagittal T1-weighted post-gadolinium MRI of hypothalamic glioma.

gical resection is in the circumstance of disfiguring proptosis or severe visual loss occurring with a tumour confined to the optic nerve. In this situation, en bloc excision of the involved optic nerve-associated tumour is generally curative. This is achieved by either a transcranial approach through the orbital roof or via a lateral orbitotomy, depending on the precise location and extent of the tumour.

For chiasmatic–hypothalamic gliomas, surgery, irradiation and chemotherapy have all been applied as either primary or adjuvant therapy.[19–24] A surgical debulking procedure carried out through a variety of transcranial approaches has proven beneficial in some circumstances; visual improvement, reduction of ICP and amelioration of hydrocephalus have all been observed, sometimes with involution of the residual tumour.[20–23] By delaying the time to disease progression, surgical intervention may also postpone the need for immediate radiation therapy—an issue important in the young child.[20] Furthermore, surgical therapy appears to have a definite beneficial role in the management of recurrent post-irradiation tumours. The devastating neuroendocrine and developmental consequences of cranial radiation in young children notwithstanding, radiation therapy does appear to have a beneficial anti-tumour affect for these lesions. In one recent report, radiation therapy increased the median time to tumour progression by 40 months and led to clinical and radiological improvement in 45% of patients.[21] Chemotherapy is emerging as an increasingly used option in young children in whom there is a desire to defer the deleterious effects of radiation. In one report, actinomycin D and vincristine induced remission in almost 63% of patients during a median follow-up of 4.3 years.[22] In a number of these, tumour shrinkage was also demonstrated. More recently, Petronio and colleagues, using several nitrosurea-based cytotoxic regimens, induced clinical remission, stabilization/improvement in visual and neurological deficits, and tumour shrinkage in up to 88% of patients during a median follow-up period of 18 months.[24] Chemotherapy may also have a role in the management of recurrent post-irradiation tumours. The overall 5-year survival rate of patients with chiasmatic–hypothalamic gliomas has been variably reported between 40% to 88%.[23]

Hamartomas (gangliocytomas) of the sellar region

Tumour-like lesions composed of neurones can, on rare occasions, present as symptomatic masses in the sellar region.[25–28] Although the nomenclature of these lesions has been confusing, including designations such as hamartoma, gangliocytoma and choristoma, the basic lesions in all cases are the same: mature neurones of varying size clustered among axons and astroglial elements. Because of their benign nature, uniformly slow growth and histological resemblance to fully differentiated hypothalamic tissue they are generally considered hamartomatous in nature. In some instances, the neuronal elements of these lesions secrete hypophysiotrophic factors, producing a clinically manifest hypersecretory state. Hamartomas of the sellar region are distinguished according to their state of origin. Those arising in the hypothalamus are referred to as hypothalamic neuronal hamartomas, whereas those arising within the sella are designated as adenohypophyseal neuronal choristomas.

Hypothalamic neuronal hamartomas

When carefully sought, ectopic foci of hypothalamic tissue are not unusual as autopsy findings, appearing as minute, macroscopic masses attached to the ventral hypothalamus, the adjacent pia or on the surface of the proximal posterior cerebral arteries. Although such hamartomatous nodules are clinically insignificant, on rare occasion they may be several centimetres in size, extend into the third ventricle, descend into the sellae, or hang in the interpeduncular cistern producing a variety of compressive and endocrinological effects. Most symptomatic examples occur in young males in whom precocious puberty is the best-known manifestation.[25] The latter features may simply be the result of hypothalamic compression; however, in some instances these lesions are found to contain gonadotrophin-releasing hormone (GnRH), thus providing an endocrine basis for accelerated sexual maturation. Other hypothalalmic neuronal hamartomas liberate growth hormone-releasing hormone (GHRH), which may induce GH cell hyperplasia and GH adenomas in the pituitary, with acromegaly being the clinical result.[26,27] Aside from other features, hypothalamic hamartomas are associated with a peculiar form of epilepsy—one characterized by laughing fits (gelastic seizures).

As a rule, hypothalamic hamartomas are generally quiescent lesions; however, others may be slowly progressive, causing visual and neurological deficits and death. Given their eloquent hypothalamic origins, the management of these lesions is often difficult. Establishing a histological diagnosis is an important initial objective, thus excluding inflammatory conditions and other tumours which may be radiosensitive (germinomas, possibly gliomas). Large masses are often amenable to significant surgical debulking—a procedure generally reserved for those lesions having documented radiological or clinical progression, and one which occasionally provides marked symptomatic benefit.

Adenohypophyseal neuronal choristoma

This lesion is histologically similar to the hypothalamic variant, but has a primary intrasellar origin, lacks anatomical continuity with the hypothalamus, and is almost invariably associated with a hypersecretory pituitary adenoma. The basic lesion consists of neurones and associated neuropil interspersed within the substance of a pituitary adenoma. It has been proposed that by way of paracrine mechanisms, choristomas release hypothalamic trophic hormones which may induce a change in adjacent adenohypophyseal cells. Of reported cases, most have occurred in the context of acromegaly, wherein the neuronal choristoma contains GHRH, and is associated with a GH-producing pituitary adenoma.[27] Similar lesions producing corticotroph-releasing hormone (CRH) have also been associated with corticotroph adenomas in the context of Cushing's disease.[28]

Because of their near-uniform association with a hypersecretory state, adenophyophyseal neuronal choristomas are always pre-operatively mistaken for functioning pituitary macroadenomas, both clinically and radiographically. Their diagnosis is revealed only after pathological examination of the surgical specimen. Given the limited number of cases reported, the long-term outcome of these lesions is uncertain, but is likely to be comparable to that of the hypersecretory tumours with which they are associated.

Parasellar granular cell tumours

Although symptomatic parasellar granular cell tumours are rare, they are nonetheless the most common primary tumour of the neurohypophysis. Historically, these lesions have been subject to a confusing terminology, one in which 'choristoma', 'granular cell myoblastoma' and 'pituicytoma' have been so variably and inconsistently applied that such nomenclature has lost any specific meaning. As incidental autopsy findings, minute granular cell tumours or 'tumourlets' are seen with surprising regularity, being present in up to 17% of carefully studied adult autopsy pituitary glands.[29] Barely visible macroscopically, these tumourlets assume the form of cryptic aggregates, often multiple, and equally distributed between the infundibulum and posterior lobe. That such incidental granular cell tumours are rarely present post mortem in individuals less than 20 years of age suggests them to be acquired lesions. The most likely progenitor of these tumours is the pituicyte—a glial element which is the dominant cell type of the neuro-hypophysis.

Symptomatic granular cell tumours are rare. Of the more than 30 or so cases reported, the majority have occurred during the fourth and fifth decades of life.[30] Most symptomatic granular cell tumours arise from the infundibulum and present as suprasellar masses. Less frequently, others take their origin from the posterior pituitary, causing sellar enlargement and eventual extension to the suprasellar region. Although globular growth in an upward direction is the rule, para- and retrosellar extensions are occasionally encountered. Rarely, granular cell tumours wholly situated within the third ventricle have been reported. The clinical presentation is non-specific; visual loss, hypopituitarism, increased ICP and diabetes insipidus are all features attributable to the tumour's compressive effects. With CT scanning, these lesions appear as large, globular, well-demarcated, homogeneously enhancing suprasellar masses. Sellar enlargement may be a feature of those tumours originating below the diaphragma. In those studied by angiography, a vascular blush is characteristically present. Given their globular, well-demarcated nature and vascularity, a granular cell tumour may mimic a suprasellar meningioma.

Large suprasellar granular cell tumours unaccompanied by sellar enlargement are approached transcranially, usually by a subfrontal or pterional approach. Intra-operatively, they appear as firm, pale masses, often with a rubbery texture. As a rule, granular cell tumours are not invasive of surrounding brain, although they are occasionally strongly adherent to it. Given their marked vascularity, heavy bleeding can usually be anticipated during the course of tumour removal. The surgical objective is chiasmal and hypothalamic decompression, although gross total resection may be attempted if it can be easily and safely accomplished. The presence of a ballooned sella in association with a granular cell tumour indicates a tumour of subdiaphragmatic origin. Accordingly, these lesions are best approached trans-sphenoidally.

The prognosis for granular cell tumours is generally favourable, with subtotal resection generally providing long-term cure. Symptomatic recurrences, although uncommon, are managed with repeat resection. Radiation therapy is unnecessary.[30]

Miscellaneous tumours of the sellar region

In addition to the major forms of sellar and parasellar neoplasia reviewed above, a variety of other rare and occasionally exotic tumours periodically involve the sellar region (Table 10.1). Despite the diversity of tumour types represented, most have a fairly non-specific clinical profile, characterized by a radiologically evident sellar/parasellar mass in association with visual dysfunction, low-grade hyperprolactinaemia and/or varying hypo-pituitarism. Given their rarity, these tumours are seldom considered in the pre-operative differential diagnosis, for most are managed as if they were seemingly ordinary endocrinologically inactive pituitary adenomas. With their true identity being revealed only after pathological examination of the surgical specimen, their diagnosis often arrives as something of a surprise.

Schwannomas

Nerve sheath tumours, although accounting for almost 10% of all intra-cranial tumours, rarely occur in the sellar and parasellar regions. In fact, only four such cases have been reported to date, with two arising from within the sellar proper showing suprasellar extension, one arising from the tuberculum sellae with suprasellar extension, and one originating from the extracavernous trigeminal nerve which also extended into the suprasellar space.[31] Schwannomas which are not seen to arise from a cranial nerve, such as those of intrasellar origin, are presumed to arise from ectopic Schwann cell rests or from autonomic vasomotor fibres. With the evolution of cavernous sinus surgery, schwannomas arising from cranial neves within the cavernous sinus are increasingly recognized and surgically managed. In a recent review by Sekhar et al, approximately 12% of 103 benign cavernous sinus tumours were schwannomas.[32] Because secondary intrasellar extension is not ordi-narily a feature of schwannomas originating in the cavernous sinus, they are readily distinguished from primary intrasellar tumours.

Paragangliomas

Paragangliomas are tumours of neural crest origin, the majority of which arise in the adrenal medulla and paraganglia. More than 80% of extra-adrenal cases involve the head and neck, with the carotid body, temporal bone and vagal body being the classical and most common sites. Though rare, there have been periodic reports of paragangliomas arising in the parasellar region. As reviewed by Steel et al, four cases have been reported to date;[33] one was of intrasellar origin, and the remaining three appeared to have arisen in the cavernous sinus and secondarily involved the sella. Headache, hypopituitarism and diplopia were variably present, with a size-able sellar region mass being a uniform finding. Two cases were approached transsphenoidally and two required a transcranial approach, with subtotal resection being achieved in all. Three of these cases were treated with post-operative radiation therapy. Given that neither the pituitary gland nor adjacent parasellar structures contain paraganglionic tissue, the cellular origins of these tumours is obscure. Persistent embryonic 'rests' of para-ganglionic tissue and/or abnormal migration of neural crest cells into the parasellar region have been invoked as possible mechanisms accounting for their origin in or around the sella.

Haemangioblastomas

Isolated accounts of sellar region haemangioblastomas, both sporadic and in association with the von Hippel–Lindau syndrome, have appeared in the literature.[34,35] In one instance the mass was entirely suprasellar, taking origin high up on the pituitary stalk.

Lipomas

Rarely, incidental lipomas of the hypothalamus are seen at autopsy, appear-ing as discrete pedunculated masses hanging down from the tuber cinereum. Genuine symptomatic examples are exceptional, and tend not only to be more adherent to, but also have parenchymal involvement with, the hypo-thalamic, tuber cinereum and mamillary bodies. Depending on their size, hypothalamic dysfunction, hyperprolactinaemia and varying degrees of hypopituitarism may all be presenting features. Although benign and slow growing, symptomatic lipomas are often so intimately related to surrounding nervous tissue that complete resection is seldom possible.[36]

Other tumours

An additional spectrum of rare and peculiar tumours of the parasellar region are the subjects of isolated case reports. These include: fibroma,[37] glom-angioma,[38] cavernous haemangioma,[39] primary melanoma,[40] myxoma,[41] osteogenic sarcoma[49] and pseudotumour.[42]

UNCOMMON OSSEOUS LESIONS OF THE SKULL BASE

In addition to chordomas (discussed above), a number of variably aggressive osseous lesions are known to involve the skull base. Their relevance to parasellar pathology derives from their occasional tendency to involve the sphenoid bone and bony sella, resulting in neurological, ophthalmological and occasionally endocrine dysfunction.

Fibrous dysplasia

Fibrous dysplasia is a non-neoplastic, developmental abnormality of bone characterized by the gradual replacement of normal bone by an abnormal fibro-osseous proliferation.[43] Generally presenting during childhood, fibrous dysplasia may progress slowly during the first three decades of life. Thereafter, the process spontaneously stops and active lesions can no longer be detected. The disorder has, by convention, been distinguished into three forms, depending on the extent of bony involvement: monostotic, polyostotic, and lesions occurring in the context of Albright's syndrome (polyostotic fibrous dysplasia, short stature, pigmented cutaneous lesions and precocious puberty, occurring most commonly in females). Craniofacial involvement may be a feature of any of these, although most skull base lesions are of the monostotic variety.

The aetiology of this disorder is unknown. The pathogenesis of fibrous dysplasia, as inferred from its histopathology, suggests the process to begin wiht proliferation of fibrous tissue in which irregularly arranged bony spicules are embedded. The lack of osteoblastic activity prevents conversion to lamellar bone, even after many years. At the skull base, involved bones undergo exuberant thickening, leading to displacement of surrounding structures and foraminal encroachment. Intraosseous haemorrhage with cystic degeneration is commonly observed. Malignant transformation (osteosarcoma, chondrosarcoma, fibrosarcoma) is exceedingly rare: most reported cases have occurred in previously irradiated lesions.[43] Depending on the relative proportion of bone, soft fibrous tissue and cystic areas, the process may manifest radiologically as sclerotic, cystic or a mixture of the two. In the skull base series of Derome, the relative proportion of each was 50%, 15% and 35%, respectively.[44]

Cranial involvement most commonly affects the frontal, ethmoid and sphenoid bones. The most common presenting feature is progressive orbito-cranial swelling, which not infrequently assumes enormous proportions, producing very significant craniofacial deformity. Proptosis and secondary exposure keratitis, restriction in globe mobility and diplopia are common accompanying features. The most important concern with this condition is blindness—a process occurring as the result of compression of the optic nerve from a thickened optic canal or, less commonly, the ischaemic result of ophthalmic artery compression. Depending on the extent of the disease, visual loss may be bilateral. In most instances, the visual deterioration is slowly progressive; however, the occasional and dramatic occurrence of sudden blindness is a well-known and worrisome feature of the condition.[44,45] Encroachment upon other cranial nerve foramina may produce additional cranial palsies. Unexplained is the association of fibrous dysplasia with a number of endocrinological conditions, including hyperthyroidism, acromegaly and Cushing's disease.[43]

CT scanning (Fig. 10.5), like skull X-rays, reveals obliteration of the

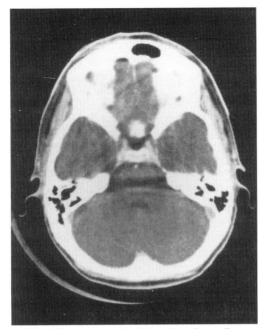

Fig. 10.5 Transverse CT of fibrous dysplasia of the tuberculum sellae.

medullary canal of involved bone by an expansile homogeneous matrix which is denser than that of normal bone, but occasionally contains focal sclerotic and lytic areas. Optic canal compromise is usually obvious. Basal and en plaque meningiomas occasionally show similar findings, although they can now be differentiated by MRI. Three-dimensional reconstructed images are indispensable when extensive craniofacial corrective procedures are anticipated. Because involved bone is typically very vascular, pre-operative angiography/embolization is often helpful.

Beyond cosmetic considerations, which are often of foremost concern to the patient, additional issues surrounding the management of fibrous dysplasia include: (1) the non-neoplastic nature of the condition; (2) the self-limiting nature of the process, which rarely progresses beyond age 30; and (3) the ominous concern of progressive or sudden visual loss. Visual loss from foraminal encroachment or threatened globe viability as the result of severe proptosis are generally considered absolute indications for surgical management. In this situation, the optic canal and/or orbit are decompressed with the removal of all involved bone. Depending on the degree of craniofacial abnormality, elaborate reconstructive procedures may also be necessary. In patients without neuro-ophthalmologic symptomatology, no treatment is generally required as virtually all cases will eventually stabilize spontaneously. Derome, in addressing the unpredictable occurrence of sudden visual loss, has also advocated 'prophylactic' decompressive surgery is visually asymptomatic patients less than 25 years of age, in whom optic canal compression is demonstrated.[44] In patients for whom cosmesis is the only concern, particularly in those with extensive craniofacial deformity requiring complex craniofacial reconstruction, surgery is generally deferred until adolescence or early adulthood.

Giant cell tumours of bone

Best known for their epiphyseal origin in long bones, giant cell tumours of bone only rarely involve the cranial vault. Of the exceptional cases which do, virtually all arise in the sphenoid or temporal bones. The predilection for giant cell tumours to arise here has been related to the unique embryology of the sphenoid and temporal bones. Unlike the remaining osseous components of the cranial vault, the sphenoid and temporal bones share with long bones of the skeleton an origin via endochondral bone formation. Fewer than 40 cases of giant cell tumour of the sphenoid bone have been reported, with most occurring in the third and fourth decades of life.[46,47] Beginning in the floor of the sella, these are destructive lesions which spread laterally and inferiorly as cohesive soft tissue masses. Destruction of the dorsum sellae is typically an early radiological feature—one eventually followed by destruction of the sphenoid wings, petrous apex and clivus. Headaches, visual loss and cranial nerve palsies are the most frequent presenting symptoms; pituitary insufficiency is rarely a feature. In the past, most cases were treated with surgical resection followed by radiation therapy.[46] More recently, particularly with the evolution of skull base surgery, as well as the concern of radiation-induced sarcomatous degeneration, there has been increasing emphasis on radical resection as the sole form of therapy.[47] Radiation therapy is reserved for incompletely excised and recurrent tumours, in addition to those with obvious malignant history. The prognosis is both variable and unpredictable. In some cases long-term quality survival is achieved; however, in others progressive or recurrent disease is accompanied by significant disability or death.

Chondrosarcomas

Cranial chondrosarcomas are rare tumours of adult life, and are occasionally difficult to differentiate from chordoma. Their preferred site of origin is the sphenoid bone, particularly in or near the sella turcica. Additional favoured sites include the petrous temporal bone and clivus. Most chondrosarcomas of the skull base are primary lesions, although a minority may arise from pre-existing chondromas or enchondromas of Ollier's disease and the related Maffucci's syndrome. As these tumours are slow growing, local pain of long duration is the most common, and frequently only, presenting complaint. With time, additional symptoms of mass effects, including cranial nerve palsies and occasionally pituitary dysfunction emerge. Metastases, typically to the lungs, occur primarily in high-grade tumours. Bony destruction is a uniform radiological feature; fine stippled calcification is often characteristic. CT and MRI will define the extent of the soft tissue mass. Radical surgical excision is the treatment of choice, whose curability diminishes as tumour size and grade increase. Periodic recurrence is not infrequent and often necessitates subsequent surgical procedures. Although most often used for incompletely resected, recurrent and high-grade tumours, the effectiveness of radiation therapy has yet to be established. The prognosis for these tumours is variable, with 5-year survival rates approaching 60%.[48]

EXTRACRANIAL TUMOURS OF THE HEAD SECONDARILY INVOLVING THE PARASELLAR REGION

Although primarily of interest to the head and neck surgeon, there are several extracranial skull base tumours whose tendency for intracranial extension is an occasional source of neurosurgical concern. These include the juvenile angiofibroma, aesthesioneuroblastomas and nasopharyngeal carcinomas.

Juvenile angiofibroma

The juvenile angiofibroma is an uncommon tumour which primarily affects adolescent males. Although a histologically benign tumour, and one whose growth characteristics are often expansive rather than invasive, the destruction potential of juvenile angiofibromas should not be overlooked; their capacity for aggressive local growth remains an ongoing and significant source of morbidity. Most of these tumours arise extracranially, with the medial pterygoid region being their most common site of origin. With progressive growth, they tend to involve the nose, nasopharynx, infra-temporal fossa, sphenoid bone, cavernous sinus, inferior and superior orbital fissures and middle cranial fossae. Because one of their routes of intracranial access involves superior extension through the roof of the sphenoid sinus into the sella, sellar and/or parasellar involvement is occasionally a feature of juvenile angiofibromas. Their most common presenting symptoms include recurrent nasal obstruction and epistaxis, the latter occasionally being quite dramatic. Additional symptoms include facial swelling, proptosis attendant to orbital extension, and cranial nerve palsies due to optic nerve compression and cavernous sinus involvement. Evidence of pituitary dysfunction is unusual. In addition to demonstrating and enchancing soft tissue mass involving the nasopharynx and the skull base, the classical CT finding is widening of the pterygopalatine fossa. MRI will clearly identify the extent of both intracranial and extracranial disease, and provide some indication of the vascularity of the tumour mass. Angiography is useful not only because of its classical appearance (early arterial blush with external carotid artery feeders), but also because of its therapeutic value, serving as a prelude to embolization.

Therapeutic options for angiofibromas, depending on their extent, include surgical resection, radiotherapy and chemotherapy, either alone or in combination. Surgery and radiotherapy are each sufficiently effective as primary treatment modalities so that the relative role of each is controversial.[50,51] Nevertheless, surgical resection remains the most widely used form of therapy, particularly in the case of smaller tumours where complete surgical resection alone is often curative. Larger and incompletely removed tumours are often treated with adjuvant radiotherapy. Given that these tumours arise extracranially and the bulk of the tumour resides there, most tumours are approached extracranially. Tumours with significant intracranial extension require combined craniofacial (extracranial–intracranial) approaches. Harrison, in a personal series of 44 patients, found that curative resections were achieved in 77% of patients. Recurrent tumours were often successfully treated by repeat resections.[51]

Aesthesioneuroblastomas

Aesthesioneuroblastoma, or olfactory neuroblastoma, is a rare tumour of neural crest origin which arises from olfactory epithelium. Having a peak incidence in the third decade of life and occurring most commonly in males, aesthesioblastomas usually begin high in the nasal cavity, extend into the paranasal sinuses, and eventually erode intracranially via the cribriform plate. Transgression of dura, brain invasion, intraorbital extension and cavernous sinus infiltration are potential sequelae of intracranial disease. Metastatic dissemination, usually to regional lymph nodes, lungs or bones, occurs in up to 30% of patients at some time during their course. Nasal obstruction, epistaxis, ocular symptoms and headache are the most common presenting features. More than half of all tumours are of advanced stage at the time of diagnosis. When intracranial extension is demonstrated, the recommended treatment protocol includes pre-operative radiation, pre- and post-operative chemotherapy and craniofacial resection. The 5-year survival rate is between 40% and 60%. Local recurrence is common which, in some instances, may occur a decade or more after initial therapy.[52,53]

Nasopharyngeal carcinoma

Nasopharyngeal carcinoma is an aggressive tumour with a propensity for skull base invasion. Although rare in North America, its dramatically increased incidence in China remains an epidemiological curiosity. The incidence peak of nasopharyngeal carcinomas approaches 50 years of age, with males being most commonly affected. Most nasopharyngeal carcinomas arise in the superior aspect of the nasopharynx and promptly invade the skull base, often extending intracranially through bony foramina.

Secondary involvement of the sphenoid sinus occurs commonly with occasional extension into the sella, cavernous sinus and parasellar region. The clinical presentation is usually one of pain, epistaxis, nasal obstruction and eventual cranial neuropathies (especially the trigeminal nerve). Radiation therapy is the primary mode of treatment, surgery being reserved for recurrent tumours. Depending on the radiosensitivity and degree of differentiation, 5-year survival rates range from 20% to 60%.[54]

CYSTIC LESIONS OF THE PARASELLAR REGION

Rathke's cleft cyst

Rathke's cleft cyst is an epithelial cyst apparently derived from remnants of Rathke's pouch, the embryological anlage of the anterior pituitary. At approximately week 4 of gestation, Rathke's pouch arises as a stomadeal evagination which extends cranially to form the craniopharyngeal duct, and later the anterior lobe of the pituitary gland. The eventual obliteration of the craniopharyngeal duct is normally accompanied by involution of Rathke's pouch. In some pituitary glands, however, discontinuous cystic remnants of the pouch may persist within the pars intermedia—the interface between the anterior and posterior lobes of the gland. Such cystic remnants, usually only of microscopic dimensions, are readily identified in up to 25% of autopsy pituitaries as incidental, clinically significant findings.[55] Occasionally such cysts, presumably by way of progressive accumulation of colloidal material, attain sufficient size to be of clinical relevance. When symptomatic, such cysts usually manifest between the third and fifth decades, and a slight female preponderance has consistently been noted.

Most symptomatic Rathke's cleft cysts arise within and remain confined to the sella turcica, causing sellar enlargement and compression of the pituitary gland and stalk.[56] An additional third of cases will exhibit significant suprasellar extension, causing visual loss, hypothalamic dysfunction and, if sufficiently large, hydrocephalus. On rare occasions pure suprasellar Rathke's cleft cysts have also been documented.[57,58] Local compressive effects are the usual basis for presentation in symptomatic cases, with headache, partial hypopituitarism, low-grade hyperprolactinaemia, visual disturbance and rarely diabetes insipidus being the principal clinical features. Unusual complications include chemical meningitis arising from the leakage of irritative cyst contents into the CSF, and infection with abscess formation. The radiological appearance of Rathke's cleft cysts is characteristic. Sellar enlargement is a common feature, except in those wholly suprasellar in location. On CT scanning most, but not all, appear as homogeneous, non-calcified, low-density, non-enhancing lesions. Their MR signal characteristics are variable, depending on the composition and consistency of their fluid contents. Nonetheless, in most instances a presumptive diagnosis of Rathke's cleft cyst can be made on radiological grounds. The difficulty arises in the occasional case having a heterogeneous fluid content, particularly one in which cellular debris is abundant. In such cases the imaging characteristics may resemble craniopharyngioma or other suprasellar tumours. It is of great practical importance to distinguish Rathke's cleft cysts from other tumours, particularly craniopharyngiomas, because the therapeutic strategies are quite different. Such distinctions can sometimes be made only by gross inspection at the time of surgery or by biopsy.

Symptomatic Rathke's cleft cysts are treated by surgical decompression.[56,59] Once a diagnosis of craniopharyngioma or other tumour has been excluded with a biopsy of the cyst wall, simple drainage with conservative, partial resection of the cyst wall will usually effect cure. Because most patients so treated have dramatic resolution of symptoms and less than 10% will recur, more aggressive surgical approaches are unjustified. With regard to surgical approach, most of the lesions can be efficiently treated via a transcranial route. A transsphenoidal approach is generally considered only for those few lesions having a wholly suprasellar disposition, where the sella is unlikely to be enlarged.

Epidermoid tumour (cyst)

Epidermoid cysts account for less than 1% of all intracranial tumours. Presumed to be products of disordered embryogenesis, epidermoid cysts arise from the aberrant inclusion of epithelial tissue or 'rests' at the time of neural tube closure or cerebral vesicle formation. Their predilection for basal brain areas and their ability to permeate along cisternal pathways account for the fact that approximately one-third of all intracranial epidermoids involve the supra- and parasellar regions. Despite their embryonic origins, few epidermoids are symptomatic before middle age.

Grossly, epidermoid cysts appear as glistening, 'pearly' white, encapsulated lesions having a waxy texture and a friable, flaky consistency. Their growth is slow—a process involving progressive desquamation of capsular elements, and the accumulation of keratin and cholesterol debris. Displacing rather than invading anatomical structures, parasellar epidermoid cysts are frequently seen to encase chiasmatic, cranial nerve and basal arterial structures, and are often tenaciously adherent to the same. Although pure intrasellar epidermoid cysts have been reported,[60] most epidermoids having a sellar component do so as the result of secondary extension from a contiguous supra- or parasellar lesion.

When symptomatic, headaches and visual dysfunction are their most common symptoms; endocrine abnormalities occur much less frequently, and hydrocephalus is rare. Because parasellar epidermoids tend to embed themselves into the mesial temporal lobe, partial complex seizures are an occasional accompaniment. The major complications of epidermoid cysts are chemical meningitis as the result of leakage of irritative cyst contents into the CSF, and the very rare phenomenon of malignant transformation into squamous cell carcinoma.[61]

The treatment of symptomatic parasellar epidermoid cysts is operative. The surgical objective is to decompress the optic apparatus and other compromised structures, removing as much tumour as is safely possible. Although a substantial portion of these cysts is easily removed, fragments densely adherent to neural and vascular structures should be left. Regrowth of residual fragments is so slow that symptomatic recurrence is infrequent. Although pure intrasellar epidermoid cysts, including those having a suprasellar component, can be approached transsphenoidally, the majority of epidermoids in this location, because of their frequent and often extensive lateral extensions, are approached transcranially.

Dermoid tumour (cyst)

Occurring with one-tenth the frequency of epidermoid cysts, dermoid cysts are rare. Given their affinity for midline intracranial sites, their occasional occurrence in the sellar and parasellar regions is well recognized, although published reports of such cases have been few.[62] In addition to the epidermal elements present in epidermoid cysts, dermoid cysts have the additional features of hair follicles, sweat and sebaceous glands. These lesions typically have a firm, fibrous capsule which is often densely adherent to surrounding structures.

Dermoid cysts tend to occur in younger patients, with most cases occurring within the first two decades of life. Their clinical presentation in the sellar region is variable, as diabetes insipidus, visual dysfunction, precocious puberty and mild hyperprolactinaemia have all been associated with dermoid cysts in this area. Some are confined exclusively to the sella, others are exclusively suprasellar, and some involve both sites. Radiologically, dermoid cysts appear as inhomogeneously enhancing masses, sometimes calcified, and often containing fat.

Like epidermoid cysts, dermoid cysts are also prone to spontaneous bouts of chemical meningitis due to seepage of their irritative cyst contents into the CSF, and they too may, very rarely, undergo malignant transformation to squamous cell carcinoma. As a rule, dermoid cysts grow more quickly than epidermoid cysts and tend to recur more frequently.

Therapy for parasellar dermoid cysts is surgical removal. Although complete surgical excision of these lesions is always desirable, their frequent adherence to cranial nerves and blood vessels often necessitates a safer, subtotal resection. Post-operative radiotherapy has not shown any benefit in either shrinking residual tumour or forestalling recurrence, and as such is not recommended. Fortunately, subtotal resection alone usually provides long-term symptom-free survival.

Arachnoid cysts

Although uncommon, arachnoid cysts do periodically arise in the region of the sella turcica, serving as an occasional source of neurological and endocrinological dysfunction in both paediatric and adult age groups. With 15% of all arachnoid cysts occurring in the sellar region, this site represents the second most common intracranial location for such lesions. Arachnoid cysts are presumed to be developmental in origin, arising as the consequence of splitting or duplication of the arachnoid membrane, forming an arachnoid lined sac in which CSF is entrapped. The natural history of these lesions remains uncertain, with some arachnoid cysts remaining quiescent for years, and others demonstrating symptomatic enlargement. The basis for such enlargement is similarly uncertain, with osmotic gradients, endogenous CSF production and progressive accumulation of CSF through a 'ball-valve' mechanism all being invoked as potential growth mechanisms. Although most arachnoid cysts are topologically related to a normal subarachnoid cistern, macroscopic continuity with the subarachnoid space is rarely apparent. Arachnoid cysts of the sellar region are distinguished as being one of two types: intrasellar and suprasellar; each is discussed separately.

Intrasellar arachnoid cysts are the least common of the two, arising from arachnoid remnants within the sella.[63] In contrast to arachnoid cysts occurring elsewhere, intrasellar arachnoid cysts tend to occur in older patients, usually in the fourth or fifth decade of life. They behave as expansile intrasellar masses, causing headache, sellar enlargement, hypopituitarism, moderate hyperprolactinaemia, and upward displacement of the diaphragma sellae, resulting in visual loss. An important anatomical feature of these lesions is that even with large suprasellar extensions the diaphragma is always intact, and the cysts remain entirely subdiaphragmatic. In rare instances, a pinhole communication with the suprasellar subarachnoid space is noted; however, as evidenced by their failure to admit contrast agents delivered cisternally, most intrasellar arachnoid cysts lack free communication with the subarachnoid space. Radiologically, these lesions are associated with sellar enlargement, appearing as homogeneous cysts whose fluid contents exhibit density and signal characteristics identical to CSF (Fig. 10.6). Intrasellar arachnoid cysts are to be distinguished from the intrasellar herniation of the chiasmatic cistern that occurs with the empty sella syndrome, and other cystic pathologies which occur in the region (craniopharyngioma, Rathke's cleft cyst, cystic pituitary adenoma, epidermoids, dermoids). Symptomatic intrasellar arachnoid cysts, as well as those in which imaging studies fail to exclude a cystic neoplasm, are best managed by transsphenoidal exploration, excision of the cyst wall for diagnosis, and marsupialization of the cyst cavity. Symptomatic improvement is the rule, headache, visual function and hyperprolactinaemia virtually always; however, anterior pituitary deficits, particularly if longstanding, are generally less responsive to surgical decompression.

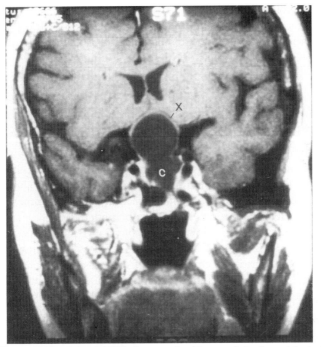

Fig. 10.6 Coronal T1-weighted MRI of an arachnoid cyst of the fossa (c) stretching and thinning the optic chiasm upwards (X).

Suprasellar arachnoid cysts are predominantly lesions of the paediatric population, with the majority of patients presenting within the first two decades of life.[23,64] Arising with the chiasmatic cistern, suprasellar arachnoid cysts may become sizeable, causing compression of the hypothalamus and third ventricle, stretching of the optic nerve and distortion of the pituitary stalk. Lateral and posterior extensions into the medial temporal lobe and interpeduncular cistern, respectively, may also occur. Hydrocephalus, on the basis of third ventricular compression or aqueductal distortion, is often the dominant presenting feature, resulting in headache, macrocephaly and retardation; precocious puberty or hypopituitarism reflects hypothalamic and/or stalk compression. Visual field deficits and loss of acuity are often present. A peculiar and intermittent pattern of head movements dubbed the 'bobble-head doll' syndrome is a rare but classical presentation of arachnoid cysts in this location.

The management of suprasellar arachnoid cysts is surgical; however, the optimal form of intervention remains a matter of debate. Marsupialization of the cyst wall, with or without some form of shunting procedure, is the principal therapeutic option; ventricoperitoneal shunting alone rarely produces a satisfactory or durable response.[23,64] Access to the cyst wall for purposes of marsupialization can be accomplished by a variety of approaches, including subfrontal, transcortical–transventricular, trans-sylvian or transcallosal routes. Once a wide excision of the cyst wall has been achieved, some authors advocate the routine placement of a cys-toperitoneal or ventriculoperitoneal shunt as marsupialization alone may fail to improve hydrocephalus, despite seemingly adequate decompression of the cyst.[23]

Empty sella syndrome

The term 'empty sella' refers to the anatomical state occurring as the result of intrasellar herniation of the subarachnoid space through an incompetent and enlarged diaphragma sellae. The result is a compressed and posteriorly displaced pituitary gland housed within an enlarged and demineralized sella. These features lend a seemingly 'empty' appearance to the sella, both grossly and radiographically. It is clinical, pathophysiological and occasionally of therapeutic importance to distinguish those cases occurring without an identifiable caue ('primary' empty sella) from those arising as the result of loss of intrasellar volume, as may accompany infarction, surgical resection or radionecrosis of an intrasellar tumour ('secondary' empty sella).

Primary empty sella syndrome

Though frequently considered the simple consequence of a developmentally enlarged diaphragmatic aperture, the primary empty sella syndrome is in fact a far more complex condition, in which diaphragmatic defects probably represent only one of several incompletely understood pathophysiological components. Autopsy studies have repeatedly shown that anatomical defects of the diaphragma sellae of 5 mm or more are present in almost 40% of consecutive autopsies, with more than 20% exhibiting intrasellar extension of the subarachnoid space,[65] and 5% showing a fully developed empty sella.[66] Insofar as the majority of these findings are incidental autopsy findings in persons without neurological or endocrine symptoms, it is likely that additional factors contribute to the development of the clinical syndrome. One potentially important contributing factor is elevated intracranial pres-sure. ICP elevations have been documented in patients with the empty sella syndrome, and at least 10% of patients with benign intracranial hypertension also have a coexisting empty sella.[67] The latter relationship is especially intriguing in that both syndromes share overlapping clinical profiles.

The overwhelming majority of patients with primary empty sella syn-drome are asymptomatic, with their empty sellae being an incidental radio-graphic finding typically discovered during the investigation of an unrelated complaint. Of the minority of patients who are symptomatic, their clinical profile is often characteristic. More than 80% of symptomatic patients are middle-aged women, many of whom are obese, multiparous and hyper-tensive.[68] Longstanding headache is the most common and frequently the only presenting complaint. Only very rarely are visual field deficits attributable to this syndrome, as symptomatic compression or intrasellar prolapse of the optic chiasm rarely occurs. Complaints of blurred vision or ophthalmological findings such as papilloedema, decreased acuity, enlarged blind spot and optic atrophy are likely to be the result of coexisting intracranial hypertension. Isolated accounts of atypical facial pain and sensory loss in the distribution of the trigeminal nerve have been noted. Clinically apparent pituitary dysfunction is unusual, although instances of pituitary deficiency, ranging from subtle abnormalities on dynamic endocrine testing (blunted GH response to insulin-induced hypoglycaemia) to rare cases of panhypopituitarism, have periodically been reported.[68,69] Moderate hyperprolactinaemia, as the result of stalk compression, has been variably reported in approximately 5% of patients.[70] Hypersecretion of other anterior pituitary hormones suggests a coexisting pituitary adenoma. Finally, CSF rhinorrhoea is a complication of empty sella syndrome in approximately 10% of patients.[69,71] As the result of CSF pulsations, the sella floor becomes progressively thinned, eventually providing communication between the intrasellar subarachnoid space and the sphenoid sinus.

The radiological diagnosis of this entity is usually straightforward. Lateral skull X-rays reveal symmetrically enlarged and thin-walled sella, one which retains its normal configuration. Both CT and MRI scanning shows clearly the CSF space traverse from the hypothalamus down to a flattened pituitary gland, a finding which virtually excludes the possibility of other cystic lesions. If the diagnosis is still in doubt, CT cisternography will demonstrate filling of the sella and conclusively secure a diagnosis of empty sella syndrome.

Secondary empty sella syndrome

This entity is the occasional consequence of prior surgical therapy or radionecrosis of an intrasellar tumour. Occasionally, the condition may occur long after auto-infarction of a pituitary adenoma or a non-tumorous pituitary gland, as may occur with apoplexy and Sheehan's syndrome, respectively. The diaphragma may be either developmentally deficient, eroded by the tumour, or disrupted by therapeutic intervention, thus permitting the descent of the chiasmatic cistern into the sella. Intrasellar prolapse of the optic chiasm is a frequent accompaniment, wherein it becomes entrapped and kinked by adhesions and scar tissue.

Clinically, the secondary empty sella syndrome is distinct from the primary form. Both sexes are equally affected and there is no predilection for any particular body habitus. Visual dysfunction is the most common presenting symptom, and may occur weeks or even years following surgery or radiotherapy. Bitemporal and binasal hemianopic defects, as well as asymmetrical deficits in the form of constrictions, segmental defects or scotomas, may occur. The visual loss is often progressive; however, abrupt deterioration has also been known to occur. Endocrine dysfunction is not unusual and is likely to be the residual effect of prior surgery and/or radiation for an intrasellar tumour, and not the result of secondary empty sella. Elevated ICP, headache and CSF rhinorrhoea are occasional features of this condition.

Treatment

Relatively few patients with primary or secondary empty sella syndrome will require surgical intervention. After establishing the diagnosis and excluding other intrasellar cystic pathologies, the management of these conditions rests primarily on the recognition and treatment of potential complications (endocrine, ophthamological and CSF rhinorrhoea). The endocrine status of the patient requires careful laboratory evaluation, both at the time of diagnosis and periodically thereafter. Hypopituitarism, if present, requires appropriate hormone replacement therapy. Except for the case of low-grade hyperprolactinaemia, hormonal hypersecretion warrants the exclusion of a hypersecreting microadenoma with MRI alone; however, when radiologically occult GH, adrenocorticotrophic hormone or prolactin-secreting microadenomas are suspected, transsphenoidal exploration may be necessary. Low-grade hyperprolactinaemia (of stalk compression origin), because of its long-term adverse affects, should be treated if associated with symptoms of hypogonadism, such as amenorrhoea, and is often exquisitely responsive to low-dose dopamine agonist therapy.

Deteriorating visual function necessitates careful evaluation. In the case of primary empty sella syndrome, this is usually the result of benign intracranial hypertension. Accordingly, appropriate therapy for the latter should be initiated. Progressive documented visual loss in the case of the secondary empty sella syndrome is usually the result of chiasmal prolapse, the extent of which can be assessed with MRI. In such cases, transsphenoidal exploration and elevation of the chiasm with fat or muscle ('chiasmopexy') may halt progression of visual loss, and in some instances may actually improve vision.[72]

CSF rhinorrhoea, because it seldom stops spontanously, will virtually always require definitive operative repair. The usual cause is a transsellar fistula into the sphenoid sinus; however, occasionally, the site of leak may be along the anterior fossa floor. Accordingly, pre-operative radiological visualization of the precise site of leak is always desirable. This is best achieved by high-resolution coronal CT cisternography. For transsellar leaks, transsphenoidal exploration, sealing of the leak with fibrin glue, and packing of the sella and sphenoid sinus with fat or fascia constitutes the treatment of choice. Leaks from the anterior fossa floor require repair by frontal craniotomy. Transnasal endoscopic methods are sometimes useful for the repair of such leaks.

METASTATIC TUMOURS TO THE SELLAR REGION

Metastatic deposits emanating from a variety of systemic and haemopoietic malignancies occasionally involve the sellar region. A favoured anatomical target for such deposits is the posterior lobe of the pituitary. The predilection of metastic tumours for the posterior lobe of the pituitary relates to its blood suppy. In contrast to the anterior pituitary, which has a somewhat tenuous and indirect supply from the portal circulation, the posterior lobe derives its circulation directly from the carotid arterial system. Although the majority of metastic tumours to this region occur in the context of advanced malignancy, occasional posterior lobe metastases may be the first sign of an unrecognized neoplastic process.[73] Of the metastic cancers, breast is the most common culpable primary, followed by lung and prostate.[74] Haemopoietic malignancies which may present with a posterior lobe deposit include the solitary plasmacytoma (Fig. 10.7) (which usually evolves into multiple myeloma),[73,75] as well as various lymphomas and leukaemias. Diabetes insipidus is often an accompanying feature, and its presence in association with a sellar mass should raise the possibility of a metastatic tumour. Additional symptoms include headache, visual field defects, hypopituitarism and cranial nerve palsies related to cavernous sinus infiltration. With the exception of diabetes insipidus, which is rarely a feature of pituitary adenoma, it is often impossible in the absence of a known history of malignancy to distinguish a metastatic tumour to the sella from a pituitary adenoma. Transsphenoidal sellar explortion and decompression will provide the tissue diagnosis and often effect symptomatic improvement, and is therefore the treatment of choice in appropriate patients. Adjuvant radiation therapy is usually required post-operatively. Depending on the responsiveness of the primary tumour and the clinical status of the patient, chemotherapy may also be considered.

INFLAMMATORY DISEASES OF THE SELLAR REGION

The sellar region is host to a diverse collection of inflammatory disorders, the pathogenesis of which can range from acute suppuration through chronic granulomatous infiltration to autoimmune processes. Only in a minority of cases is the presenting clinical or radiological appearance suggestive of the pathological diagnosis; in most cases, their inflammatory basis is revealed only after careful pathological examination of the surgical specimen.

Infections

Pituitary abscess

Acute bacterial infection of the sella turcica is a rare event, with only 50 or so documented cases in the literature.[77] Although in most instances the pathogenesis of pituitary infection is not apparent, studies in which an

(a)

(b)

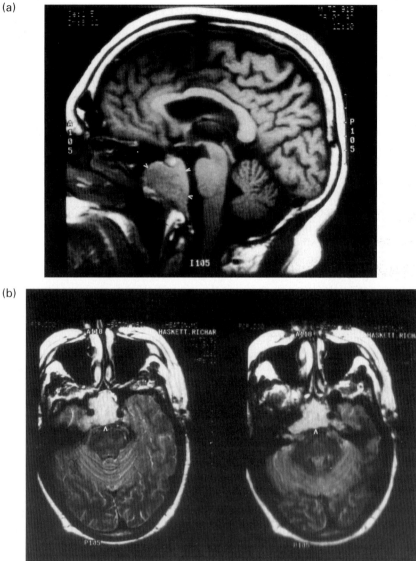

Fig. 10.7 (a) Saggittal and (b) two consecutive transverse T1 MRI scans of a plasmocytoma (white arrowheads) centred on the clivus.

aetiology has been established suggest that pituitary abscess arises in two clinical settings. The first appears to be the result of secondary extension from a pre-existing, anatomically contiguous purulent focus. Acute sphenoid sinusitis, osteomyelitis of the sphenoid bone, mastoiditis, cavernous sinus thrombophlebitis, peritonsillar abscess, purulent otitis media and bacterial meningitis have all been implicated as the primary infectious source. The other principal pathogenetic mechanism relates to generalized sepsis and haematogenous dissemination from a variety of distant septic foci (pneumonia, osteomyelitis, endocarditis, retroperitoneal abscess). Isolated pituitary abscesses are extremely rare. More commonly (although still extremely unusual) abscesses have been reported in association with pre-existing sellar lesions (pituitary adenoma, craniopharyngioma, Rathke's cyst).[77] Why such lesions should be especially vulnerable to abscess formation is unclear.

The symptoms of pituitary abscess are non-specific, and frequently indistinguishable from those of other sellar mass lesions (headache, visual field deficits, hypopituitarism). However, when these symptoms are accompanied by features of meningitis, the possibility of a pituitary abscess should be strongly considered. As reviewed by Domingue and Wilson, most patients will have some radiological evidence of sellar pathology, the result of either a pre-existing lesion or of the abscess itself. The bacteriology of pituitary abscess is variable. When organisms have been isolated, *Staphylococcus aureus, Diplococcus pneumoniae*, group A *Streptococcus, Klebsiella* species, *Escherichia coli* and *Citrobacter divercusis* are most frequently reported.[77]

The management of a suspected pituitary abscess includes transsphenoidal exploration of the sella, drainage of the inflammatory mass and antibiotic therapy. Selection of antimicrobial agents is based ideally on culture reports; however, when organisms cannot be isolated, or a responsible primary infectious source is not identified, broad-spectrum therapy is indicated. The combination of a third-generation cephalosporin, a synthetic penicillin and metronidazole for their Gram-negative, staphylococcal and anaerobic sensitivities, respectively, is a suitable choice. The optimal duration of antibiotic therapy has not been established.

Because of their rarity, recent data concerning the long-term outcome for pituitary abscesses are not available. Based on their review of 29 cases, Domingue and Wilson identified an overall mortality rate of 28% for pituitary abscess, which further increased to 45% if meningitis was also present.[77]

Miscellaneous infections

A variety of other rare non-bacterial infective agents may also be responsible for pituitary and sellar region infection. Tuberculosis, still endemic in certain areas, has historically been an important aetiology for destructive, granulomatous inflammatory lesions involving the hypothalamus and sellar region.[79] In most instances, parasellar involvement has been a complication of its dense, plaque-like basilar meningitis. Such 'tuberculomas' are often associated with near-total anterior and posterior pituitary failure, are frequently calcified and often, but not invariably, associated with evidence of active tuberculosis elsewhere.

Syphilis, now extremely uncommon in its consummate forms, represents another granulomatous infection involving the hypothalamus and sellar region.[80] Historical accounts suggest that the clinical features of syphilitic gumma in the sellar region were typical of other destructive processes of the sella, and were usually associated with syphilitic lesions elsewhere in the neuroaxis.

Mycotic infection, notably aspergillosis, has also been reported to involve the sellar, parasellar and orbital regions, often presenting as a discrete inflammatory mass.[81] Parasitic infiltration of the sellar and parapituitary regions by cystcercosis[82] and echinococcus[83] have both been known to produce a mass in this region. Finally, in the context of AIDS and other immunosuppressed states, an additional spectrum of pituitary infection has emerged, including agents such as *Pneumocystis carinii, Toxoplasma gondii* and cytomegalovirus.[84]

Mucoceles

Mucoceles are benign, slowly expansile, mucous-filled cystic lesions which arise in paranasal sinuses. Their neurosurgical relevance derives primarily from their very occasional tendency to erode intracranially, wherein they may present as an intracranial mass or, less frequently, offer a source for intracranial infection. While mucoceles arising in the maxillary sinus are numerically the most frequent, and those arising in the frontal and anterior ethmoid sinuses are clinically the most significant, this discussion concerns those rare mucoceles arising from the sphenoid or posterior ethmoid sinuses, whose intracranial involvement brings them into the realm of parasellar pathology.

Mucoceles of the sphenoid and posterior ethmoid sinuses (sphenoethmoid mucoceles) are rare. Rarer still is the occasion when these mucoceles erode through the sellar floor and present as intrasellar, parasellar or suprasellar masses.[85-87] In some instances their clinical features are indistinguishable from those of a non-functioning pituitary adenoma; the sella is eroded, showing balloon-like enlargement, and a chiasmal syndrome attendant to suprasellar extension is documented. In other cases there may be more extensive intracranial involvement, with extensions into the orbital apex and superior orbital fissure. In such cases additional symptoms of exophthalmos and oculomotor palsies may also be present. Hypopituitarism is rarely a feature of sellar region mucoceles. On CT scanning most mucoceles will appear isodense, although their walls may exhibit contrast enhancement of varying degree. Bone windows will reveal the extent of bony erosion and/or destruction. Their MRI signal characteristics are variable, depending on the viscosity of contents.

Pathologically, mucoceles are encapsulated masses whose walls are composed of the mucoperiosteal lining of the involved sinus. Their pathogenesis remains conjectural. Although post-inflammatory obstruction of the sinus

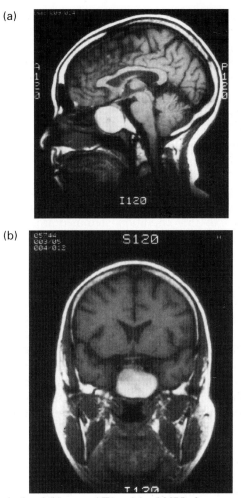

Fig. 10.8 (**a**) Saggittal and (**b**) coronal T1-weighted MRI of a mucopyocele of the sphenoid sinus.

ostia is the most commonly invoked mechanism underlying their development, mucoceles appear to be neither a common nor inevitable result of such obstruction. Whatever the basis for their initiation, mucoceles are generally chronic lesions, frequently exhibiting years of subclinical growth before causing symptoms. Ongoing accumulation of mucoid material gives rise to expansile growth, causing bony erosion of the sinus walls, and eventual access to the intracranial compartment. Mucoceles which become infected are known as 'mucopyoceles' and, expectedly, have an abruptly accelerated course, often with rapid bony destruction and an increased risk of intracranial or intraoribtal infection (Fig. 10.8).

Sphenoidoethmoidal mucoceles are effectively treated by transsphenoidal or transethmoidal exploration, depending on their sinus of origin. Drainage of mucocele contents and mucosal exenteration of the involved sinus is generally curative. Radical removal of the intracranial portion of the muco-cele wall is neither necessary nor advisable.[85]

Non-infectious inflammatory lesions of the sellar region

Lymphocytic hypophysitis

Lymphocytic hypophysitis is a destructive, inflammatory disorder of the anterior pituitary, presumed to be autoimmune in origin. Although the earliest descriptions of this condition stemmed from necropsy studies wherein the potentially lethal nature of the disorder was emphasized, improved recognition of the condition coupled with hormone replacement therapy have since rendered lymphocytic hypophysitis an entirely treatable condition.

The basic lesion consists of a destructive, inflammatory infiltrate of lym-phocytes, plasma cells and macrophages which is restricted exclusively to the anterior lobe of the gland. The result is a firm and enlarged gland which often extends into the suprasellar space, and microscopically exhibits effacement of the normal glandular architecture and disruption of the struc-tural and immunohistochemical integrity of all anterior lobe secretory elements.[88] Lymphoid follicles and loosely organized germinal centres may be present, as are varying degrees of fibrosis, depending on the chronicity of the condition. Several lines of evidence suggest this process to have an autoimmune basis.[89-91] Firstly, the cellular infiltrate present in affected glands is similar to other autoimmune reactions occurring in other organs. Anti-pituitary antibodies have been indentified in the serum of some patients with the condition. Finally, patients with lymphocytic hypophysitis not infrequently have a concurrent or prior history of other autoimmune diseases (Hashimoto's thyroiditis, idiopathic adrenalitis, pancreatitis and others), thus suggesting that lymphocytic hypophysitis is but one component of a generalized polyglandular autoimmune disorder.

The clinical profile of lymphocytic hypophysitis is fairly characteristic.[88-91] While the condition was once believed to affect women exclusively, ever-increasing reports of its occurrence in men have established that males too may be affected, although considerably less often. One of the most typical features of the condition concerns its temporal association with pregnancy; almost 70% of reported cases occur during pregnancy or more commonly during the first postpartum year. Indeed the condition is sometimes called post-partum hypophysitis. Clinically, the picture is one of progressive anterior pituitary failure in association with an expansile sellar mass. The pituitary insufficiency may involve any or all anterior pituitary hormones;

manifestations of hypocorticolism have been especially prominent among reported cases. Amenorrhoea or failure of appropriate resumption of menses following parturition is a common presenting complaint; galactorrhoea occurs less frequently. The amenorrhoea is at least in part related to the moderate hyperprolactinaemia which is a result of pituitary stalk compression, a common accompaniment to the condition. Because the posterior lobe escapes injury, diabetes insipidus is not ordinarily a feature of the condition. Since there is often considerable enlargement of the gland, the majority of patients will also have symptoms of mass effect, including headache and visual loss. The radiological appearance of lymphocytic hypophysitis is non-specific. Plain films may demonstrate sellar enlargement, contrast CT scanning reveals a densely enhancing sellar mass, often with suprasellar extension, and MRI scanning shows a sellar/suprasellar mass which is homogeneously isointense to brain parenchyma.

In its most typical clinical context, such as that involving the pregnant or post-partum female presenting with a sellar region mass, lymphocytic hypophysitis should be an obvious diagnostic consideration. Prolactin-producing pituitary adenomas, given their known tendency to enlarge during pregnancy, are probably the most commonly considered differential diagnosis. In other clinical situations not related to pregnancy, or those involving male patients, a prospective diagnosis of a lymphocytic hypophysitis cannot be made with any certainty. In all cases, however, the definitive diagnosis requires histological confirmation. Accordingly, the management of this condition involves establishing a tissue diagnosis and chiasmal decompression—objectives best served by the transsphenoidal route. The gland typically appears very firm, diffusely enlarged and has a pale yellow appearance. The surgical goal is to remove sufficient tissue for histological diagnosis and chiasmal decompression while preserving as much of the viable gland as possible, thus maximizing prospects for residual pituitary function.

Given the presumed autoimmune origins of lymphocytic hypophysitis, the therapeutic use of immunosuppressive agents has met with some success as an adjuvant form of therapy for this condition. In some patients, corticosteroid therapy has resulted in reduction in the size of the sellar mass and improvement in visual function, prompting some authors to recommend such therapy from the start, thus avoiding the immediate need for surgical decompression or tissue diagnosis.[90] It is to be acknowledged, however, that experience with this approach has been limited and that steroids have not proven uniformly successful in ameliorating the inflammatory process.[92]

Endocrine replacement therapy is an essential component of the management of this disorder. Pituitary insufficiency should be carefully assessed and appropriately treated both at presentation and during long-term follow-up. Because the degree of anterior pituitary destruction is typically quite severe, most patients with lymphocytic hypophysitis will require chronic long-term replacement therapy.

Sarcoidosis

Known as one of the 'great imitators', sarcoidosis is well recognized for its periodic affinity for parasellar structures, serving as an occasional diagnosis of exclusion for masses and other inflammatory processes affecting this region.[93] As a chronic, multi-system, granulomatous disease of unknown origin, sarcoidosis can affect any organ or tissue, with uveoparotitis, pulmonary and lymph node involvement being its classical manifestations. Five per cent of all cases will exhibit nervous system involvement, most commonly in the form of dense adhesive granulomatous arachnoiditis involving the base of the brain.[94] Cranial nerves, the pituitary gland stalk, hypothalamic and anterior third ventricular structures may all be engulfed in the inflammatory process. Less frequently, neurosarcoidosis can assume the form of discrete masses, both in the parasellar region and elsewhere in the neuroaxis.

The clinical features of neurosarcoidosis are variable and reflect the degree of anatomical involvement. The hypothalamus and pituitary stalk are favoured targets, and accordingly features of hypothalamic dysfunction often predominate.[93-96] The single most common feature of CNS involvement— one occasionally serving as the presenting feature of the disease in general— is diabetes insipidus. This usually reflects hypothalamic involvement and, less often, damage to the stalk. Additional evidence of hypothalamic disease in the form of somnolence and alterations of eating, emotion and thermoregulation often coexist. Damage to hypophysiotropic areas of the hypothalamus or the stalk can result in hypopituitarism and low-grade hyperprolactinaemia. Primary involvement of the anterior pituitary may also be the source of hypopituitarism, but less commonly. Visual dysfunction secondary to optic nerve and chiasmal involvement also occurs. Depending on the extent of basilar meningeal involvement, other cranial nerve palsies may also occur. Hydrocephalus, reflecting basilar meningeal or third ventricular obstruction, may be present.

Imaging studies, when positive, generally reveal an enhancing meningeal process, or evidence of a discrete mass of the sellar region. A search for active disease in the lungs or elsewhere is often informative in providing corroborative evidence of sarcoidosis; however, definite diagnosis requires biopsy. Because the histopathology of sarcoidosis is often characteristic, but falls short of being diagnostic, this is a diagnosis of exclusion. A compatible clinical profile, histological evidence of non-caseating granulomas, and negative bacterial and fungal cultures of biopsy specimens are the practical diagnostic criteria used for this entity. CSF studies, though frequently abnormal (lymphocytic pleocytosis, elevations of protein and immunoglobins, decreased glucose concentrations), are non-specific.

From the surgical perspective most, if not all, cases of sarcoidosis involving the sellar region will present as undiagnosed mass lesions, occurring in the absence of recognized systemic sarcoidosis. Therefore the surgical objectives primarily include establishing a tissue diagnosis and decompression of the visual apparatus. Once the diagnosis is established, corticosteroids are often effective therapy. In cases unresponsive to steroids, chloroquine, aza-thioprine and methotrexate have all been used with varying degrees of success. The prognosis is variable, being most favourable in patients with limited disease, where spontaneous remission is also occasionally seen.[97] In other patients, particularly those with pulmonary involvement and disease in more than three organ systems, the prognosis is poor.

Langerhans cell histiocytosis (histiocytosis X)

Langerhans cell histiocytosis is an umbrella term encompassing a collection of poorly understood, clinically heterogeneous but pathologically inter-related entities. Unified pathologically and pathognomonically by a destructive infiltrate of foamy histiocytes in affected organs, the clinical expression of Langerhans cell histiocytes is variable, depending on the extent and nature of organ involvement. Ranging from the fulminant, disseminated and frequently fatal Letterer–Siwe disease seen in childhood, through the multifocal eosinophilic granulomas of Hand–Schuller–Christian disease, and to the relatively innocent solitary eosinophilic granulomas of bone, involvement of parasellar structures may be a feature of each.[98]

CNS involvement, usually in association with multifocal bony lesions, occurs in almost one-quarter of all patients with systemic Langerhans cell histiocytosis; isolated CNS involvement is, however, rare.[99] There is an apparent predilection for involvement of the hypothalamus, infundibulum and posterior pituitary, with adenohypophyseal involvement occurring less frequently.[98–102] In some cases the disease is discretely localized in the hypothalamus or posterior pituitary. In other cases the process is less restricted, with bony disease of the skull base and secondary infiltrates both compressing and permeating meningeal and multiple parasellar structures. Diabetes insipidus is the most common presenting feature of CNS disease, and not uncommonly is the first sign of unrecognized systemic disease. Hyperprolactinaemia on the basis of stalk or hypothalamic involvement may also present. Involvement of the optic apparatus occurs less frequently, and anterior pituitary function is often spared. Imaging studies are non-specific, typically revealing obvious bony disease, with a contiguous soft tissue component.

If the diagnosis is already known, due to the multisystem nature of the disease, there is no role for surgical intervention. In the rare situation of an isolated parasellar granuloma, the surgical objective in this condition is directed primarily at establishing a histological diagnosis, and possibly decompression of compromised sellar structures. A definitive diagnosis rests on the identification of the intracytoplasmic organelles known as Birbeck granules, the demonstration that cells of the histiocytic infiltrate bear the CD1 antigenic determinant, and the confirmation that bacterial and fungal cultures of the surgical specimen are negative. The role of radiotherapy remains uncertain, as are the roles for chemotherapy and immunotherapy in progressive systemic or intracranial disease, as discussed by Dunger et al in 1991.

ANEURYSMS OF THE SELLAR REGION

Although uncommon, the possibility of a cerebral aneurysm masquerading as a pituitary adenoma has always been an important, if not a nagging diagnostic consideration in the evaluation of an endocrine-inactive sellar mass. Indeed, the inadvertent rupture of an unsuspected intrasellar aneurysm during the course of transsphenoidal exploration for a presumed pituitary adenoma represents one of the classical neurosurgical disasters.[103] That cerebral angiography was, until recently, a regular practice in the radiological evaluation of pituitary adenomas further emphasizes the fact that aneurysms do periodically involve the sellar region, and their exclusion is essential. Fortunately, one of the many benefits of MRI is its ability to exclude an aneurysm as a potential aetiology of a sellar region mass, thus obviating the routine use of angiography. The majority of aneurysms involving the sellar region derive from the intracavernous segment of the carotid artery, and less often from the supraclinoid carotid and the anterior communicating artery complex. The clinical picture may be indistinguishable from a non-functioning pituitary adenoma or other sellar mass; headache and retro-orbital pain, visual symptoms, low-grade hyperprolactinaemia and, less commonly, hypopituitarism and diabetes insipidus have all been reported as presenting features. Should such aneurysms erode into and occupy the sella, the resulting sellar enlargement can be indistinguishable from that occurring with pituitary adenomas or other intrasellar mass lesions.

In addition to mimicking pituitary adenomas, aneurysms have also been known to coexist with pituitary adenomas. As reviewed by Weir, the incidence of coexisting pituitary adenomas and incidental cerebral aneurysms approaches 7.4% in various reports.[104] GH-producing pituitary tumours in particular have been repeatedly reported to coexist with incidental aneurysms at a frequency above what would be expected by chance alone. The basis of this association is uncertain. Because generalized arterial ectasia is a recognized feature of acromegaly, some have speculated that the local effects of GH or, more likely, of insulin-like growth factor 1 (IGF-1) on cerebral blood vessels (which are known to have IGF-1 receptors) may in some way predispose or contribute to aneurysm formation.

REFERENCES

1. Laws ER Jr. Craniopharyngioma: diagnosis and treatment. Endocrinologist, 1992; 184–188.

2. Laws ER Jr. Craniopharyngiomas: diagnosis and treatment. In: Sekhar LN, Schramm VL (eds) Tumors of the cranial base: diagnosis and treatment. Mount Kisco, NY: Futura, 1987; pp 347–371.
3. Burger PC, Scheithauer BW, Vogel FS. Surgical pathology of the nervous system and its coverings (3rd ed). Edinburgh: Churchill Livingstone, 1991; pp 545.
4. Laws ER Jr. Transsphenoidal microsurgery in the management of craniopharyngiomas. J Neurosurg, 1980; 52: 661–666.
5. Coffey RL, Lunsford LD. The role of stereotactic techniques in the management of craniopharyngiomas. Neurosurg Clin North Am, 1990; 1: 161–172.
6. Baskin DS, Wilson CB. Surgical management of craniopharyngiomas: a review of 74 cases. J Neurosurg 1986; 65: 22–27.
7. Jennings MT, Gelman R, Hochberg F. Intracranial germ-cell tumors: natural history and pathogenesis. J Neurosurg 1985; 63: 155–167.
8. Baskin DS, Wilson CB. Transsphenoidal management of intrasellar germinomas. J Neurosurg 1983; 59: 1063–1066.
9. Baumgartner JE, Edwards MSB. Pineal tumors. Neurosurg Clin N Am 1992; 3: 853–862.
10. Allen JC. Controversies in the management of intracranial germ cell tumors. Neurol Clin 1991; 9: 441–452.
11. Legido A, Packer RJ, Sutton LN et al. Suprasellar germinomas of childhood: a reappraisal. Cancer 1989; 63: 340–344.
12. Horowitz MB, Hall WA. Central nervous system germinomas. Arch Neurol 1991; 48: 652–657.
13. Allen JC, Kim JH, Packer RJ. Neoadjuvant chemotherapy for newly diagnosed germ cell tumors of the central nervous system. J Neurosurg 1987; 67: 65–70.
14. Grisoli F, Vincentelli F, Raybaud C et al. Intrasellar meningioma. Surg Neurol 1983; 20: 36–41.
15. Guthrie BL, Ebersold MJ, Scheithauer BW. Neoplasms of the intracranial meninges. In: Youmans J (ed) Neurological surgery (3rd ed). Philadelphia: Saunders, 1990; pp 3250–3315.
16. Laws ER Jr. Clival chordomas. In: Sekhar LN, Janecka IP (eds) Surgery of cranial base tumors. New York: Raven Press, 1993; pp 679–686.
17. Derome PJ. The transbasal approach to tumours invading the skull base. In: Schmidek HH, Sweet WH (eds) Operative neurosurgical techniques (Vol 1). New York: Grune & Stratton, 1988; pp 619–633.
18. Black KL. Chordomas of the clival region. Contemp Neurosurg 1990; 12: 1–7.
19. Cohen ME, Duffner PK. Optic pathway tumors. Neurol Clin 1991; 9: 764–477.
20. Wisoff JH, Abbott R, Epstein F. Surgical management of exophytic chiasmatic–hypothalamic tumors of childhood. J Neurosurg 1990; 73: 661–667.
21. Rodriguez LA, Edwards MSB, Levin VA. Management of hypothalamic gliomas in children: an analysis of 33 cases. Neurosurgery 1990; 26: 242–247.
22. Packer RJ, Sutton LN, Bilaniuk LT et al. Treatment of chiasmatic/hypothalamic gliomas of childhood with chemotherapy: an update. Ann Neurol 1988; 23: 79–85.
23. Rutka JT, Hoffman HJ, Drake JM et al. Suprasellar and sellar tumors in childhood and adolescence. Neurosurg Clin North Am 1992; 3: 803–820.
24. Petronio J, Edwards MSB, Prados M et al. Management of chiasmal and hypothalamic gliomas of infancy and childhood with chemotherapy. J Neurosurg 1991; 74: 701–708.
25. Albright AL, Lee PA. Neurosurgical treatment of hypothalamic hamartomas causing precocious puberty. J Neurosurg 1993; 78: 77–82.
26. Asa SL, Bilbao JM, Kovacs K, Linfoot JA. Hypothalamic neuronal hamartoma associated with pituitary growth hormone cell adenoma and acromegaly. Acta Neuropathol (Berl) 1980; 52: 231–234.
27. Scheithauer BW, Kovacs K, Randall RV et al. Hypothalamic neuronal hamartoma and adenohypophyseal neuronal choristoma: their association with growth hormone adenomas of the pituitary gland. J Neuropathol Exp Neurol 1983; 42: 648–663.
28. Asa SL, Kovacs K, Tindall GT et al. Cushing's disease associated with an intrasellar gangliocytoma producing corticotropin-releasing factor. Ann Intern Med 1984; 100: 789–793.
29. Luse SA, Kernohan JW. Granular cell tumors of the stalk and posterior lobe of the pituitary gland. Cancer 1955; 8: 616–622.

30. Becker DH, Wilson CB. Symptomatic parasellar granular cell tumors. Neurosurgery 1981; 8: 173–180.
31. Wilberger JE. Primary intrasellar schwannoma: case report. Surg Neurol 1989; 32: 156–158.
32. Sekhar LN, Ross DA, Sen C. Cavernous sinus and sphenocavernous neoplasms: anatomy and surgery. In: Sekhar LN, Janecka IP (eds) Surgery of cranial base tumors. New York: Raven Press, 1993; pp 603.
33. Steel TR, Daily AT, Born D et al. Paragangliomas of the sellar region: report of two cases. Neurosurgery 1993; 32: 844–847.
34. Dan NG, Smith DE. Pituitary hemangioblastoma in a patient with von Hippel–Lindau disease. J Neurosurg 1975; 42: 232–235.
35. Grisoli F, Gambarelli D, Raybaud C et al. Suprasellar hemangioblastoma. Surg Neurol 1984; 22: 257–262.
36. Kazner E, Stochdorph O, Wende S et al. Intracranial lipoma: diagnostic and therapeutic considerations. J Neurosurg 1980; 52: 234–245.
37. Frank E, Derauz J-P, de Tribolet N. Chondromyxoid fibroma of the petrous–sphenoid junction. Surg Neurol 1987; 27: 182–186.
38. Asa SL, Kovacs K, Horvath E et al. Sellar glomangioma. Ultrastruct Pathol 1984; 7: 49–54.
39. Sansone ME, Liwnicz BH, Mandybur TI. Giant pituitary cavernous hemangioma. J Neurosurg 1980; 53: 124–126.
40. Scholtz CL, Siu K. Melanoma of the pituitary. J Neurosurg 1976; 45: 101–103.
41. Nagatani M, Mori S, Takimoto N et al. Primary myxoma in the pituitary fossa: case report. Neurosurgery 1987; 20: 329–331.
42. Gartman JJ, Powers SK, Fortune M. Pseudotumor of the sellar and parasellar areas. Neurosurgery 1989; 24: 896–901.
43. Krane SM, Schiller AL. Hyperostosis, neoplasms, and other disorders of bone and cartilage. In: Petersdorf RG, Adams RD, Braunwald E et al (eds) Harrison's principles of internal medicine (10th ed). New York: McGraw-Hill, 1983; pp 1968–1969.
44. Derome P, Visot A. Bony lesions of the anterior and middle cranial fossa. In: Sekhar LN, Schramm VL (eds) Tumors of the cranial base: diagnosis and treatment. Mount Kisco, NY: Futura, 1987; pp 304–307.
45. Weisman JS, Helper RS, Vinters HV. Reversible visual loss caused by fibrous dysplasia. Am J Ophthalmol 1990; 110: 244–249.
46. Wolfe JT, Scheithauer BW, Dahlin DC. Giant cell tumor of the sphenoid bone; review of 10 cases. J Neurosurg 1983; 59: 322–327.
47. Watkins LD, Uttley D, Archer DJ et al. Giant cell tumors of the sphenoid bone. Neurosurgery 1992; 30: 576–581.
48. Stapleton SR, Wilkins PR, Archer DJ, Uttley D. Chondrosarcoma of the skull base: a series of eight cases. Neurosurgery 1993; 32: 348–356.
49. Reichenthal E, Cohen ML, Manor R et al. Primary osteogenic sarcoma of the sellar region. J Neurosurg 1981; 55: 299–302.
50. Cummings BJ, Blend R, Keane T et al. Primary radiation therapy for juvenile nasopharyngeal angiofibroma. Laryngoscope 1984; 94: 1599–1605.
51. Harrison DF. The natural history, pathogenesis, and treatment of juvenile nasopharyngeal angiofibroma. Arch Otolaryngol Head Neck Surg 1987; 113: 936–941.
52. Cantrell RW. Esthesioneuroblastoma. In: Sekhar LN, Janecka IP (eds) Surgery of cranial base tumors. New York: Raven Press, 1993; pp 471–476.
53. Levine PA, McLean WC, Cantrell RW. Esthesioneuroblastoma: the University of Virginia experience 1960–1985. Laryngoscope 1986; 96: 742–746.
54. Synderman CH, Sekhar LN, Sen CN, Janecka IP. Malignant skull base tumors. Neurosurg Clin N Am 1990; 1: 243–259.
55. Kovacs K, Horvath E. Tumors of the pituitary gland. In: Atlas of tumor pathology (fascicle 21, 2nd series). Washington DC: Armed Forces Institute of Pathology, 1986; pp 1–269.
56. Baskin DS, Wilson CB. Transsphenoidal treatment of non-neoplastic intrasellar cysts: a report of 38 cases. J Neurosurg 1984; 60: 8–13.
57. Barrow DL, Spector RH, Takei Y, Tindall GT. Symptomatic Rathke's cleft cysts located entirely in the suprasellar region: review of diagnosis, management, and pathogenesis. Neurosurgery 1985; 16: 766–772.

58. Itoh J, Usui K. An entirely suprasellar symptomatic Rathke's cleft cyst: case report. Neurosurgery 1992; 30: 581–585.
59. Midha R, Jay V, Smyth HS. Transsphenoidal management of Rathke's cleft cysts: a clinicopathological review of 10 cases. Surg Neurol 1991; 35: 446–454.
60. Boggan JE, Davis RL, Zorman G, Wilson CB. Intrasellar epidermoid cyst: case report. J Neurosurg 1983; 58: 411–415.
61. Lewis AJ, Cooper PW, Kassel EE, Schwartz ML. Squamous cell carcinoma arising in a suprasellar epidermoid cyst: case report. J Neurosurg 1983; 59: 538–541.
62. Klonoff DC, Kahn DG, Rosenzweig W, Wilson CB. Hyperprolactinemia in a patient with a pituitary and ovarian dermoid tumor: case report. Neurosurgery 1990; 26: 335–339.
63. Meyer FB, Carpenter SM, Laws ER Jr. Intrasellar arachnoid cysts. Surg Neurol 1987; 28: 105–110.
64. Jones RFC, Warnock TH, Nayanar V, Gupta JM. Suprasellar arachnoid cysts: management by cyst wall resection. Neurosurgery 1989; 25: 554–561.
65. Bergland RM, Ray BS, Torack RM. Anatomical variations in the pituitary gland and adjacent structures in 225 human autopsy cases. J Neurosurg 1968; 28: 93–99.
66. Kaufman B, Chamberlin WB Jr. The ubiquitous 'empty' sella turcica. Acta Radiol Diagn (Stockholm) 1972; 13: 413–425.
67. Weisberg LA, Housepian EM, Saur DP. Empty sella syndrome as a complication of benign intracranial hypertension. J Neurosurg 1975; 43: 177–180.
68. Neelon FA, Goree JA, Lebovitz HE. The primary empty sella: clinical and radiographic characteristics and endocrine function. Medicine 1973; 52: 73–92.
69. Gharib H, Frey HM, Laws ER Jr et al. Co-existent primary empty sella syndrome and hyperprolactinemia: report of 11 cases. Arch Intern Med 1983; 143: 1383–1386.
70. Weisberg LA, Zimmerman EA, Frantz A. Diagnosis and evaluation of patients with an enlarged sella turcica. Am J Med 1976; 61: 590–596.
71. Applebaum EL, Desai NM. Primary empty sella syndrome with CSF rhinorrhea. JAMA 1980; 244: 1606–1608.
72. Welch K, Stears JC. Chiasmapexy for the correction of traction on the optic nerves and chiasm associated with their descent into an empty sella turcica: case report. J Neurosurg 1971; 35: 760–764.
73. Branch CL, Laws ER Jr. Metastatic tumors of the sella turcica masquerading as primary pituitary tumors. J Clin Endocrinol Metab 1987; 65: 649–474.
74. Teears RJ, Silverman EM. Clinicopathologic review of 88 cases of carcinoma metastatic to the pituitary gland. Cancer 1975; 36: 216–222.
75. Dhanani A-NN, Bilbao JM, Kovacs K. Multiple myeloma presenting as a sellar plasmacytoma and mimicking a pituitary tumor: report of a case and review of the literature. Endocr Pathol 1990; 1: 245–248.
76. Berger SA, Edberg SC, David G. Infectious disease in the sella turcica. Rev Infect Dis 1986; 8: 747–755.
77. Domingue JN, Wilson CB. Pituitary abscesses: report of seven cases and review of the literature. J Neurosurg 1977; 46: 601–608.
78. Lindholm J, Rassmussen P, Korsgaard O. Intrasellar or pituitary abscess. J Neurosurg 1973; 38: 616–619.
79. Udani PM, Parekh UC, Dastur DK. Neurological and related syndromes in CNS tuberculosis. J Neurol Sci 1971; 14: 341–357.
80. Oelbaum MH. Hypopituitarism in male subjects due to syphilis. Q J Med 1952; 45: 249–266.
81. Ramos-Gabatin A, Jordan RM. Primary pituitary aspergillosis responding to transsphenoidal surgery and combined therapy with amphotericin-B and 5-fluorocytosine: case report. J Neurosurg 1981; 54: 839–841.
82. Del Brutto OH, Guevara J, Sotelo J. Intrasellar cysticercosis. J Neurosurg 1988; 69: 58–60.
83. Osgen T, Bertan V, Kansu T et al. Intrasellar hydatid cyst: case report. J Neurosurg 1984; 60: 647–648.
84. Sano T, Kovacs K, Scheithauer BW et al. Pituitary pathology in acquired immunodeficiency syndrome. Arch Pathol Lab Med 1989; 113: 1066–1070.
85. Abla A, Maroon JC, Wilberger JE et al. Intrasellar mucocele simulating a pituitary adenoma: case report. Neurosurgery 1986; 18: 197–199.

86. Close NG, O'Conner WE. Sphenoethmoidal mucoceles with intracranial extension. Otolaryngol Head Neck Surg 1983; 91: 350–357.
87. Delfini R, Missori P, Ianerri G et al. Mucoceles of the paranasal sinuses with intracranial and intraorbital extension: report of 28 cases. Neurosurgery 1993; 32: 901–906.
88. Asa SL, Bilbao JM, Kovacs K et al. Lymphocytic hypophysitis of pregnancy resulting in hypopituitarism: a distinct clinicopathologic entity. Ann Intern Med 1981; 95: 166–171.
89. Thorner ML, Vance ML, Horvath E, Kovacs K. The anterior pituitary. In: Wilson JD, Foster DW (eds) Williams textbook of endocrinology (8th ed). Philadelphia: Saunders, 1992; pp 221–310.
90. Feigenbaum SL, Martin MC, Wilson CB, Jaffe RB. Lymphocytic adenohypophysitis: a pituitary mass lesion occurring in pregnancy. Proposal for medical treatment. Am J Obstet Gynecol 1991; 164: 1549–1555.
91. Cosman F, Post KD, Holub DA, Wardlaw SL. Lymphocytic hypophysitis: report of 3 new cases and review of the literature. Medicine 1989; 68: 240–256.
92. Reusch JEB, Kleinschmidt-DeMasters BK, Lillehei KO et al. Preoperative diagnosis of lymphocytic hypophysitis (adenohypophysitis) unresponsive to short course dexamethasone: case report. Neurosurgery 1992; 30: 268–272.
93. Capellan JIL, Olmedo C, Martin JM et al. Intrasellar mass with hypopituitarism as a manifestation of sarcoidosis. J Neurosurg 1990; 73: 283–286.
94. Stern BJ, Krumholz A, Johns C et al. Sarcoidosis and its neurological manifestations. Arch Neurol 1985; 42: 909–917.
95. Pentland B, Mitchell JD, Cull RE, Ford MJ. Central nervous system sarcoidosis. Q J Med 1985; 56: 457–465.
96. Scott IA, Stocks AE, Saines N. Hypothalamic/pituitary sarcoidosis. Aust NZ J Med 1987; 17: 243–245.
97. Crystal RG. Sarcoidosis. In Wilson JD, Braunwald E, Isselbacher K et al (eds) Harrison's principles of internal medicine (12th ed). New York: McGraw-Hill, 1992; pp. 1463–1469.
98. Favara BE, Jaffe R. Pathology of Langerhans' cell histiocytosis. Hematol Oncol Clin North Am 1987; 1: 75–97.
99. Lieberman PH, Jones CR, Dargeon HWK, Begg CF. A re-appraisal of eosinophilic granuloma of bone, Hand–Schuller–Christian syndrome, and Letterer–Siwe syndrome. Medicine 1969; 48: 375–400.
100. Tibbs PA, Challa V, Mortara RH. Isolated histiocytosis X of the hypothalamus: case report. J Neurosurg 1978; 49: 929–934.
101. Ober KP, Alexander E, Challa VR et al. Histiocytosis X of the hypothalamus. Neurosurgery 1989; 24: 93–98.
102. Nishio S, Mizuno J, Barrow DL et al. Isolated histiocytosis X of the pituitary gland: case report. Neurosurgery 1987; 21: 718–721.
103. White JC, Ballantine HT Jr. Intrasellar aneurysm simulating hypophyseal tumors. J Neurosurg 1961; 18: 34–50.
104. Weir B. Pituitary tumors and aneurysm: case report and review of the literature. Neurosurgery 1992; 30: 585–591.

11 | Controversial issues

Stafford Lightman, Michael Powell

Where there are different ways of treating a condition, particularly if a number of different specialties are involved, there will always be areas for debate. Sometimes debate occurs within a single specialty and sometimes between specialties. In pituitary disease there are more than a few controversial issues. We present what we hope is a sane and rational but most importantly *joint* view of some of these issues.

PRIMARY DOPAMINE THERAPY IN PROLACTINOMAS

Bromocriptine and an increasing family of other dopamine agonist drugs are powerful agents in the management of prolactinoma. They cause rapid inhibition of prolactin secretion and reduction of cytoplasmic volume which results in dramatic tumour shrinkage in the majority of cases. Eventually these changes may lead to permanent tumour regression, although this may take years.

Macroprolactinomas

What are the relative merits of dopamine agonist therapy and surgery in macroadenomas? Some surgeons would still argue that the best form of treatment is surgery followed by radiotherapy, because they believe that the ideal is to have a patient who is 'normal' and off all therapy. They would also argue that there is always a chance of surgical cure, albeit small. We would disagree with this view. Surgery alone seldom cures the hyper-prolactinaemia of macroprolactinomas, most patients still requiring long-term treatment with dopamine agonists. Normal post-operative prolactin levels depend on total tumour removal, which because of the anatomical features of the fossa and cavernous sinus is technically difficult and thus rarely achieved. As surgeons are prepared to use dopamine agonists in surgically 'impossible' tumours, it is clearly illogical to offer surgery to the patients with the surgically easier tumours. Furthermore, there is always the risk, albeit small, of inducing hypopituitarism in the surgically treated patient. We believe that all patients should be treated medically and surgery reserved for the dopamine agonist non-responders.

Microprolactinomas

These seldom come directly to neurosurgeons, since for many years they have been treated very successfully with dopamine agonists. The argument against surgery has always been that apart from the perceived risk the surgery may only be temporarily curative, with a 50% recurrence at five years. This view was based largely on the report by Serri on the surgical series of Jules Hardy, the Montreal pituitary surgeon who is rightly credited as the father of modern pituitary surgery. However, this series studies prolactin levels, not functional recovery. Serri reviewed this series in 1993, and Hardy subsequently re-reviewed their even longer-term review of these patients. These same patients, between 10 and 20 years from surgery, have approximately 75% functional cure at review, although some continue to have a modestly raised prolactin. These figures are similar to a 10-year review of surgically treated microprolactinomas reported from Glasgow University.[1]

Most surgeons enjoy the experience of operating on the 'virgin' micro-prolactinoma which has not undergone any change through long-term dopamine agonist treatment. The tumours usually shell out in a very satis-factorily fashion from the normal gland, and are technically the most easy of all microadenomas to operate on, with excellent post-operative results. These are the features that make a case surgically 'satisfying' for doctor and patient alike. Conversely, prolactinomas that have undergone long-term treatment with bromocriptine are often very difficult, with tough fibrous glands in which the tumour boundaries are indistinct. Although this type of change is not universal following therapy, it certainly reduces the success rate for surgery in this group of patients.

These comments are not intended to be taken as a plea for a change of approach in the treatment of microprolactinoma. Medical management remains highly successful, but it should serve as a reminder that surgery is a credible alternative in the patient who is either intolerant to drugs, or dislikes the idea of long-term medical therapy.

INDICATIONS FOR THE PRIMARY USE OF MEDICAL THERAPY IN NON-FUNCTIONING MACROADENOMAS

In our view there is no place for medical management of these tumours. It is illogical to treat with bromocriptine a tumour that is not secreting prolactin, even if the level of prolactin is slightly raised through stalk compression. A large prolactinoma should secrete prolactin to levels in excess of 6000 mU/l. Medical therapy in non-functioning tumours will lull the clinician into a state of false security, believing that something is being 'done', particularly in the female patient whose menstrual cycle recommences.

INCIDENTALLY FOUND MACROADENOMAS AND MICROADENOMAS

With increasing freedom of access to scanning, pituitary tumours are being discovered as incidental findings, particularly during screening for other conditions. It is difficult to offer the reader an opinion based on sufficient experience; however, as most pituitary tumours are indolent in their growth rates, a watch-and-wait policy could be adopted. If the patient is endocrinologically normal, has normal vision, and is not troubled by headaches it would seem reasonable to review with time rather than leap to surgery. This strategy must be discussed carefully with the patient. It will be important to educate the patient on the development of visual dysfunction, and provide a strategy for review which will include ophthalmic assessment and repeat magnetic resonance imaging (MRI) to assess possible tumour growth.

As the quality and resolution of MRI scans has improved, it has become apparent that 'innocent' non-secreting microadenomas may be picked up when patients are scanned for small secreting adenomas, in particular corticotroph 'Cushing's' adenomas. This has increased the need for good biochemical diagnosis and localization of Cushing's disease. It reinforces the maxim that abnormalities of function *must* be sought before conclusions are drawn from abnormalities of structure. Our approach to this problem is outlined in Chapter 3.

PROLACTINOMAS AND PREGNANCY

Even normal pituitary glands increase in size during pregnancy and the same is true of most pituitary tumours. There is, however, a false perception that pituitary tumours and pregnancy are in some way incompatible. It is our own experience and that of Laws (personal communication) that pro-lactinomas do not cause untreatable problems in pregnancy regardless of size. Emergency surgery for a previously identified pituitary tumour of any type is exceptional. When a previously unidentified large tumour does present, its management should be based on the same considerations as in the non-pregnant patient, although if surgery is required the anaesthetist would, of course, need to consider any specific problems of anaesthesia during pregnancy. The medical management of pituitary tumours in preg-nancy has been set out in detail in Chapter 3.

FAILED AND 'FAILED FAILED' ENDOCRINE SURGERY

Even in the best centres, the cure rate for hypersecreting functional tumours remains below 100%. The figures from the best centres have been given in the post-operative management chapter. Optimum management would include identification of the results of surgery whilst the patient is still in hospital. If operative failure is identified early, repeat surgery can be per-formed immediately when reoperation is straightforward, particularly if the tumour was identified at the first operation, and hopefully the residual fragment can be found and removed. If time has elapsed, it is always worth repeating the MRI although the interpretation of post-operative change can, on occasion, be difficult.[2] There is considerable value in review being carried out in a multidisciplinary clinic. Discussion between surgeon, endo-crinologist and patient clarifies the treatment strategies.

Unless there were anatomical difficulties or the tumour was impossible to identify at the first operation, it is always, in our view, worth repeating the operation. Anatomical difficulties would include midline carotids, false aneurysms from previous carotid damage and invasion of the cavernous sinus. In patients whose surgery was performed elsewhere, it is quite com-mon to find that either the fossa was opened on only one side or not opened at all. It is important for the patient and surgeon to realize that second surgery has a lower success rate.

Third-time surgery is seldom curative. Surgeons should resist the temp-tation to perform a total hypophysectomy, as this seldom results in control of hormone hypersecretion and leaves the patient with panhypopituitarism and the lifelong need for hormone replacement.

Failure of surgery in hormone-secreting tumours necessitates different treatment for the three conditions. There is an absolute need to control cortisol hypersecretion in Cushing's tumours. If no further pituitary surgery is contemplated, cortisol excess must be treated with adrenalectomy. The tumour must be treated at a later date with pituitary irradiation to prevent the development of Nelson's syndrome. In failed surgery for acromegaly, it is equally important to control growth hormone hypersecretion. Radiotherapy can and usually will achieve this with time. The use of somatostatin during the time that radiotherapy is having its effect will minimize the symptoms of the condition and may decrease the cardiovascular risk of the hypersecretion. Failed prolactinoma surgery in drug-resistant or intolerant patients should be followed by radiotherapy.

There is early evidence from specialist radiotherapy centres that single-dose stereotactic radiotherapy to the tumour bed, rather than the fractionated dose treatments using either stereotactic or conventional three-port radiotherapy, may achieve more rapid control of surgery-resistant hormone-secreting tumours. Further trials are needed before these treatment techniques can be fully established.

CRANIOPHARYNGIOMAS

The management of this difficult tumour is one of the most controversial areas in pituitary management. In children, it is the commonest parasellar tumour, and one of the most common intracranial lesions. In this age group it is often aggressive, and can be difficult to control despite a combination of surgery and radiotherapy. There are considerable problems that can arise from both these therapies, particularly in the smaller child. In adults, the disease is much more indolent and seldom the killer as in children. However, the pitfalls of treatment can be just as devastating.

These tumours can appear anywhere from the floor of the fossa to the hypothalamus, and may be extremely large, filling the third and even the lateral ventricles. Located solely within the fossa, there is a better case for total removal, but even here this may not be possible, and the price is usually panhypopituitarism with diabetes insipidus.

Paediatric craniopharyngiomas may be dealt with according to the plan offered in Chapter 2. Aggressive surgery does claim some 'total' cures (as opposed to near total removal), but the recurrence rate in these series is usually significant, such as in Hoffman's series which quotes 17 in 45 children.[3] Clever approaches to the third ventricle are available, and multiple-stage operative procedures may be necessary.[4] Hydrocephalus often complicates the larger tumours, particularly in children.

In the *adult*, in whom the tumour presents with visual loss, chiasmal decompression must be carried out. This is relatively easy in tumours situated below the chiasm, either through a pterional craniotomy, or a transsphenoidal route can be used if the fossa is enlarged, particularly if the pituitary gland is not functioning. However, these tumours are often found in the retrochiasmatic region. If vision has to be saved, retrochiasmatic approaches have to be utilized, of which the sylvian fissure splitting route is probably safest. Neurosurgeons have devised a number of ingenious ways to get to these tumours, such as through the lamina terminalis and through the corpus callosum.[4] Where vision is not at risk, biopsy can be used to confirm the diagnosis and radiotherapy given if the lesion is shown to be growing. Biopsy is necessary to exclude the other parasellar lesions such as Rathke's cleft cysts, which do not require this aggressive treatment.

The price paid for surgery can be great.[5] Many of these tumours involve the hypothalamus, and quite apart from the almost inevitable panhypopituitarism and diabetes insipidus, somnolescence, hyperphagia, difficult fluid and electrolyte balance and memory and intellectual difficulties can result from enthusiastic surgery. Of these somnolescence and hyperphagia are both particularly distressing and difficult to manage. It is the family, the general practitioner, district nurses and in children special schools which often have to pick up the pieces resulting from over-ambitious surgery. Even limited surgery can result in distressing personality changes.

Radiotherapy can offer equally good remission rates, without the attendant morbidity. This particularly applies to adults and older children, although the younger child will suffer intellectual problems and growth difficulties as a result. Other strategies are available, particularly for the cystic forms, where intracyst yttrium and bleomycin both offer hope.

REFERENCES

1. Thompson JA, Davis DL, McLaren EH, Teasdale GM. Ten year follow up of microprolactinomas treated by transsphenoidal surgery. Br Med J 1994; 309: 1409–1410.
2. Dana TS, Feaster SH, Laws ER, Davis DO. Magnetic resonance of the pituitary gland post surgery: serial MR studies following transsphenoidal resection. AJR 1993; 14: 763–776.
3. Hoffman H, De Silva M, Humphreys R et al. Aggressive management of craniophariongiomas in children. J Neurosurg 1992; 76: 47–52.
4. Samii M, Cheatham ML, Becker DP. Craniopharingiomas. In: Atlas of skull base surgery. Philadelphia: Saunders, 1995: pp 176–185.
5. Fisher E, Welsh K, Schillito J et al. Craniopharingiomas in children: long term effects of conservative surgical procedures combined with radiation therapy. J Neurosurg 1990; 73: 534–540.
6. Hardy J, Serri O. Long term follow up of transsphenoidal resection of microprolactinomas, 10 to 20 years follow up. In: Brock M, Fuhrmann H, Hoell T et al, eds. Proceedings of the 10th European Congress of Neurosurgery (Abstracts). Berlin, 1995: p 48.
7. Serri O, Hardy J, Massoud F. Relapse of hyperprolactinaemia revisited. N Engl J Med 1993; 329: 1357.

Index

229